Beating
The Devil

D1743691

Simon Turner

chipmunkapublishing
the mental health publisher

Published by
Chipmunkapublishing
PO Box 6872
Brentwood
Essex CM13 1ZT
United Kingdom

http://www.chipmunkapublishing.com

Edited by Aleks Lech

Chipmunkapublishing gratefully acknowledge the support of Arts Council England.

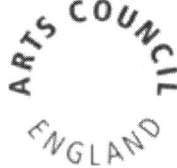

Chapter 1 - Escape to France

October 1988

Fired at forty. What the hell to do? I returned home in a state of shock. All I could think of was the utter humiliation but my long suffering wife Mandy reminded me that I now had a new opportunity to do what I really wanted to do in life at last. I still had over £75000 in cash sitting in the bank from the recent sale of our house so money wasn't an immediate problem. The immediate problem was my own mental state.

I had spent over twenty two years in 'The Property Game' before being ignominiously and finally despatched after only six months with Messrs Hamptons Estate Agents at Great Dunmow. Born with a silver spoon in my mouth this was my first professional setback in life and it hurt like hell.

Nevertheless I took my wife's advice and started to look elsewhere. Then my mother of all people recommended an article by Lesley Garner in the Daily Telegraph entitled 'Recklessness and the 40-year itch' where she wrote very percipiently:-

'Male or female, we hear the ticking of the biological clock and the rush of time's winged chariot. In front of us lies old age and oblivion. Behind lie all those things we meant to do but did not. All around lies everything we stand to lose if we get it wrong this time. Because of the confluence of pressures, the recklessness of youth is as nothing to the recklessness of middle age. Middle-aged people are much braver than the young. At 40, exquisite, pivotal moment, it is not too late. Just.'

She finished her article by writing:-

'Forty is a time to stop waffling. Either you realize your dreams or you let them go gracefully like the balloons of childhood.'

Just after reading the above article I also read that anyone can learn a foreign language if they really want to. That did it. I had been aimlessly fiddling for some time with the vague idea of buying a property in France as the prices there seemed to be at least five times cheaper than in rural Essex. I had originally been looking in the north of France in the Normandy area but soon decided that the climate was too similar to that in England and gradually worked south and west. Then I was sent some details by Shirley Temple, an English agent from near Toulouse, and at the same time a portentous article appeared in The Independent newspaper. It was entitled 'At the Sign of the Red Rocker' by the distinguished journalist and Americanist Godfrey Hodgson in which he glorified the cuisine and the way of life in Gascony.

The Fact File at the end of the article also mentioned the vital piece of information that Air France offered regular Heathrow to Toulouse flights at only £116 return for a ticket booked at least 14 days in advance.

That clinched it. I booked my flight immediately and was soon on my way. It was late November by now and Heathrow had been shrouded in a dense fog all day. The plane was delayed for over two hours and I thought it would probably be cancelled. There is something infinitely depressing about waiting round airports, especially the dingy Terminal 2 on your own, and I was beginning to get cold feet and a horrible wave of depression swept over me, along with a splitting headache. However, eventually we got the call and after an uneventful flight, landed at Blagnac Airport in the *banlieu* (outskirts) of Toulouse in the early hours. Those were the good old, mad old days when you could still smoke on a plane, on Air France at least. They always stuck us puffers in at the very back of the plane which was the safest place I always thought in case of emergency, and you usually had the bonus of a spare seat or two next to you which greatly reduced the claustrophobia. Nowadays the planes are always jam packed and one always seems to sit next to some overweight gentleman who takes up at least one and a half seats. It seems rather unfair when a slip of a girl pays a small fortune to Mr O'Leary for a mere two or three pounds excess baggage whilst the guy next to her who has stones of excess baggage round his waist but no actual travel baggage pays nothing extra at all. Well, we wouldn't want to be too sizist in today's brave new world of political correctness, would we? However there could soon be a silver lining as Air France are studying proposals to charge extra large people for two seats. Blinding.

Shirley was there at the airport to take me back to her place where she was providing bed and breakfast. It was about a forty five minute drive from the airport and I had no idea of my surroundings. All I was aware of was the almost total blackness except for a couple of small villages and a few lights twinkling in the distance. I felt very alone and disembodied.

The next day was totally different as I awoke refreshed to find brilliant sunshine and a sharp white frost. Gone were the claustrophobic grey skies of East Anglia as I found myself wandering in a winter wonderland. Shirley's house was situated near the little town of Beaumont-de-Lomagne in the Tarn and Garonne *département* about fifty kilometers north west of Toulouse. The countryside was 'delightfully undulating', to utilize a typical estate agents cliché, with great tracts of brown, bare arable land. I quickly dismissed the three specific properties I had come to see, but in the late afternoon sunshine I found the house of my dreams. And that latter word was fatefully accurate because that was exactly what it was, a dream but not reality. We had crossed the border and were now in the Gers *département* (pronounced *jairs* by the locals not the classic *jair* of snooty Parisiens), or number 32 out of the 95 departments which make up the Hexagon. My house of dreams was in the romantic sounding hamlet of Saint Martin de las Oumettes. For some time I was led to believe that las Oumettes was translated as little angels but was later to find out that actually it far more prosaically meant little elms. The property was perched on the top of a hillside almost a thousand feet above sea level and had the most incredible views over the surrounding, predominantly arable countryside, but dotted with small woods and rugged stone built farmhouses. On a clear day you could see all the way to the Pyrenees over a hundred kilometers away.

The house itself was an impressive nineteenth century *'maison de maitre'* (literally house of the master) which immediately appealed to me with my carefully retained delusions of grandeur. It was rather run down and in need of several licks of paint but to my ex- surveyor's eyes the roof seemed sound and the structure solid. It also had magnificent tiled floors, massive open fireplaces and a huge patio to enjoy the 'stunning views', to continue through the repertoire of estate agents' clichés. The temperature was still in the mid sixties as we wandered over the two arable fields that went with the property. I thought cornily and with humble apologies to William Wordsworth that:-

Bliss was it that day to be alive
But to be in the Gers was very heaven.

Back to basics. The original details that Shirley had sent me contained only pictures of the back of the house and had made me immediately dismiss it as the photos of the property were so poor they made it look like an out of place Mediterranean villa. Also the original asking price was eight hundred and fifty thousand francs which was miles over my budget of fifty thousand pounds. For the younger reader brought up on Euros the exchange rate then was approximately ten francs to the pound. However the original owner of the property had recently died and the children were apparently very keen to sell (i.e. desperate). The asking price was now down to six hundred and fifty thousand francs, definitely within striking range. Back at the office there was some very rapid foreplay between myself, Shirley and the *notaire* (solicitor) she worked for, plus the various offspring. I thought we had clinched a deal at five hundred thousand francs for the house and one of the arable fields. Unfortunately, at the subsequent signing ceremony the *notaire* tried to persuade me to buy the other field for an extra fifty thousand francs. This was above my agreed maximum and I backed off saying that I would have to return home and discuss the matter with my wife. I later found out that after I had flown off into the sunset Shirley's husband turned to her and said that it was the last they had seen of me.

But he couldn't have been more wrong. A fool and his money are soon parted. As soon as I had got home and shown the pictures to Mandy, I realized what a tremendous bargain the property was and immediately booked to fly back the next week. However this time the flight wasn't a modest one hundred and sixteen pounds return but an usurious two hundred and ninety three pounds. But as the French would at this stage say *attention*, a bargain is not a bargain if you don't need it. Of course I wasn't paying much attention and ploughed on regardless. This time there was no problem with the *sous-seeing privée* or preliminary contract and I duly signed on the dotted line. I was committed but should I have been certified as well?

Back in England I was still serving out my notice with Hamptons Estate Agents and what a lingering death it was. Everyone knew of my situation but no-one talked about it. It was as if I were suffering from the plague, or more topically swine flu. My misery was completed on my last day at the office with only one colleague taking pity upon me by buying me a modest pint at lunchtime. I slunk away about five o'clock and at six on the dot some bright spark arrived at my home to requisition my company Sierra. Goodbye to 'The Property Game'. Ah well, I tried to comfort myself that it hadn't really been my scene but inside I was still bleeding.

I had already enrolled at the Berlitz Language School off Oxford Street in London for the little matter of £5000. Why I hadn't applied at one of the numerous Cambridge equivalents which were both much nearer and cheaper I just don't know. And why didn't I enrol Mandy at the same time? But then I didn't know why I did most things at that time. You could feebly say it was written in the stars. Anyway what you could safely say was that my wife had to do all the hard work and look after our three young children at the same time while I indulged myself on my personal pet project.

I had enrolled at Berlitz on a one to one basis and what followed was the toughest two months mental work I have ever done. I used to leave in the dark for an hour's drive to Leytonstone. There I had to forego the private comforts of my motor car for the impersonal tribulations of the tube before striding down Oxford Street to the Berlitz School where my brain then had to move into overdrive. Five hours French a day for a thrice failed 'O' Level student almost twenty five years earlier was exhausting enough, although I didn't go all the way with the fiendish 'Total Immersion'. The latter not only involved over seven hours a day in the classroom but all meals and breaks with the teachers as well. There was no hiding place for me either as I was relentlessly grilled by a string of young French *professeurs*. However the latter were more than *sympathique*, especially when they found out that I was the only student there actually paying for the course with his own money and was also going to live and work in France, unlike the rest of my fellow students who were all on company duty. My teachers helped to kindle my enthusiasm for my proposed way of life with tales of

Toulouse, the beautiful *ville rose*, *cassoulet* and hot sunshine. Some of the girls were also stunningly attractive. It proved very difficult to think at all, let alone wrestle with the subjunctive in French, whilst in close proximity with Sabine's divine black stockinged legs. The maverick Jean-Claude became a close drinking companion after school as the Conservative government in all its liberal wisdom had just extended pub hours to all day opening like their continental companions. In the tavern he regaled me with the reverse perils of the English language for foreigners. Like the time he was struggling to open an unwilling bottle of wine in front of a sophisticated young couple during a stint as a waiter when he both alarmed and delighted them by revealing confidentially that 'zee cock is too hard'. I was reciprocally sympathetic when I found out that they were only been paid about four pounds an hour while I was paying the Berlitz School of Language twenty pounds an hour. With their indefatigable support I battled on and at the end of eight weeks hard labour, I found myself surprisingly proficient despite being the proud possessor of a strangely anglicised accent. However I never managed to crack the big one, actually being able to think in French which is absolutely imperative if you want to become truly proficient.

At the beginning of the course I had only a very vague idea of what I was actually going to do in France apart from to disappear off the face of the map. Oh yes, I had always been shit hot on planning. However with Jean-Claude's assistance, I gradually formulated a plan for a '*cafe-couette*' (literally cafe with duvet), or bed and breakfast establishment. However the going was still very tough and I was frequently overcome by bouts of unexplained nausea, not that I was sensible enough actually to see a doctor, let alone speak to my wife about my problem. In fact I retired hurt to my bed on Christmas Day with a splitting headache, too woebegone to even drink a glass of Veuve Cliquot. If one couldn't even face The Widow it must have been bad. However all I could feebly answer to

Mandy's increasingly desperate cries of 'What's wrong?' was 'I just don't know'. Ring any bells out there?

You might well wonder what my Irish wife and three young daughters thought about this madcap venture. I was totally oblivious at the time to Mandy waking up continually in the middle of the night in a flat panic at what I was doing. Luckily the children were too young to really understand what was going on while she was always prepared to do anything that might help me refind the joy of living. Not many wives would have gone along with this deluded, arrogant Englishman. Of course it wouldn't have made any difference what she said anyway because once I had decided to run away to France it was all over bar the shouting.

Whilst I was indulging myself at Berlitz Mandy meanwhile spent many hours with the girls with English flash cards, having carefully printed the French equivalent on the back. She told me only about this very recently. She went on to say in a very aggrieved fashion that although she had only scraped a French 'O' Level herself and her accent was appalling, the girls were at least learning to spell in French although they had no idea what was to befall them and no thanks to me.

I finished my course at Berlitz in February and it was now time for me to go back to Beaumont-de-Lomagne and sign the completion document or *acte definitive*. Shirley assured me that the weather had been wonderful for the last two months. I chose to drive down in order that I could visit some *café-couettes* on the way and get some ideas on prices and how they were run. I arrived at a wild and windy Folkestone where by one of those strange coincidences in life I bumped into Gary Hudson and his charming wife Belinda. I had played cricket with him at Bishops Stortford Cricket Club and he was one of the few friends I had made there. He was also a French teacher in real life and was on a little trip to Switzerland visiting old haunts. Our cosy little chat was soon interrupted by all and sundry retching round about us in the stormy sea just after we had left the haven of the harbour so I left the locker room for some fresh air where I just about managed to hold on to my sea legs.

We arrived in the dark in Boulogne and I hadn't realized quite how far the journey was to Amiens, my first port of call. From there I took a huge detour round Paris to Angers on the River Loire in Western Brittany and felt that now familiar feeling of nausea most of the time. On the third day I drove down to the Dordogne. The sun was shining, the roads were empty and life suddenly seemed a bit better. The *cafe-couettes* were all very pleasant but old fashioned and too formal and that wasn't what I was looking for at all. The fourth day I drove on down to the Gers. Unfortunately the weather had broken and it was very gloomy indeed as I crossed the mighty Garonne at Valence D'Agen. Suddenly I got the shock of my life when two huge chimneys emerged through the gloom. Somebody had neglected to tell me that France's newest nuclear power station was being constructed only twenty five kilometers from the house of my dreams. I don't think that the Gallic Property Descriptions Act covered these sorts of omissions or emissions either, but it ill behove a former Chartered Surveyor not to have carried out his own thorough survey of the area.

After this distinctly unpromising start I drove down the last bit of my journey to Saint Clar, thinking not that Simon was coming home but what the hell was he doing there at all. The owners had kindly consented to let me stay at Saint Martin before the actual signing, rather different to England. So off I toddled and saw the Gascon caretaker, Roger Auzeric, who was to be my dearest if not quite my nearest neighbour for the next four years. He had apparently also looked after the property for the previous owners for many years. Peter Mayle has subsequently immortalized the southern twang of '*pang*', '*chang*' and '*enfang*' etc, instead of pain, champ and enfin, but in the spring of 89 Berlitz had merely hinted at the problems I would encounter with the local patois. My other near neighbour Monsieur Magnier would also prove to be very friendly if not almost totally incomprehensible. However I did find out from his wife that we were infinitely preferable to the Pirlets, our snooty Parisien predecessors. Christ, the locals despised Parisiens, almost as much as the hated *musulman* (Moslem). Not much PC down here. Of course a lot of the farmers in this area of France were *pied noirs*, or black feet, who had been forced to flee Algeria after the War of Independence and weren't having the *musulman* following them back to France. However much, much more on this subject later on.

Roger Auzeric was a very fit and wiry sixty something and about five foot nothing in his bare feet. He had twinkling blue eyes and a typically scornful *hein* if he couldn't understand a word of my Suffolk burr, although he did kindly consent to being quite impressed by my new found fluency in the French language. He had the usual small arable farm of about forty hectares with assorted birds and animals, plus the obligatory small vineyard which provided enough wine for him and his family. He never drank coffee, let alone tea, but just had small sips of red wine from time to time during the day. He also distilled his own Armagnac which I was later to market at Auberge Saint Martin as the local 'firewater' at ten francs a throw. And very good firewater it was too.

After Roger had shown me the ropes and how the excellent central heating system worked he left me to my own devices. I unfolded my card table, unrolled my sleeping bag and shut out the dark night with the shutters. The latter are sensibly obligatory for security insurance purposes in France, as well as keeping out the heat in summer and the heat in during the winter months. Nobody had told me how cold it could get in winter but I was later to find out for myself the hard way. I found myself rattling round this vast house on my own in the middle of nowhere and it felt like a prison. However after a few glasses of the local red wine the world seemed a better place and I shuffled off to bed. Fortunately I had bought some of the bedroom furniture so had a place to lay my weary head and soon drifted off into a deep sleep. However I was woken suddenly from my slumbers by a howling gale and a dripping of water that I traced to the opposite bedroom. So much for my surveyor's roof diagnosis and dreams of unbroken sunshine.

The next day the signing at Beaumont went like clockwork with that very smooth operator *Maître* Max Miquel, the *notaire,* in the chair. I do like the French titles and Maître gives just the right amount of respect and reverence to the person in authority. However I don't think many solicitors I have met in England would deserve the accolade .

After the signing Shirley and I adjourned to the Café de Sport for an expresso coffee and an armagnac to celebrate my purchase. The next few days found me very busy organizing all the various necessities, the first and foremost being to meet the mayor of my commune at Mauroux. Monsieur Dubarry couldn't have been more charming or helpful and got me to fill in the important book of life and other formalities with his ancient secretary. The French are obsessed with bureaucracy and I was given a vast list of documents to assemble on my return to England, including my old 'A' Level and 'O' Level certificates which I hadn't seen since the Sixties. That said there is method in their madness. Indeed one improvement we have recently adopted from the continent is to have photographs on driving licences, if not their *carte d'identités* and *Carte de Séjour* (work permit) as yet. All that Anglo Saxon balls about loss of freedom makes me mad. Credit card fraud and under age drinking could be cut at a stroke if we adopted their system. However our nannying Government proposed to bring in Identity Cards for all the wrong reasons. They should be utilized exclusively for civil matters, not the absurd notion that we actually might catch terrorists with them. In fact for many years I found the simplest way of proving my identity back in England was my old *Carte de Séjour*.

Meanwhile I had been sleeping very badly back in my mausoleum and drinking increasingly enthusiastically to bury my growing feeling of unease which manifested itself physically with further increasing bouts of nausea. Therefore by the time I was ready to return to England I was virtually all in. Therefore it was with a heavy heart and an even heavier hangover that I set off on my long drive back on that fateful Tuesday morning. Roger had advised me against my better judgement to go via Montauban to the north east. However as the locals general geographical knowledge didn't extend even to the next *département*, let alone the rest of France, it proved to be a grave mistake and added literally hours to an already tortuous journey. Of course by far the quickest route would have been to take the *autoroute* via Bordeaux. After five hours driving on the wearisome old N20 behind painfully slow and smelly diesel lorries on the slopes of the Massif Central, I eventually arrived at the outskirts of Limoges at about lunchtime. The Black Prince had earned the well-deserved epithet 'The Butcher of Limoges' in 1346 during the 'The Hundred Years War' and what followed was pretty black as well. I pressed on for a little bit till I was clear of the city and then stopped for a much needed thermos of strong black coffee and an apple. Seemingly refreshed I set off again on the daunting journey to Caen. Some time later I began to feel a bit weird but gritted my teeth and battled on in the manner of a true Brit. However I soon begun to realize something was very seriously amiss. There appeared to an iron vice round my chest and I had great difficulty in breathing. I stopped in a little village for a walk and some fresh air but that only seemed to aggravate the situation as I went all dizzy and my legs felt like lead. I asked a villager if there was a doctor in the vicinity but he replied that the nearest one was in Argentan about twenty kilometers away. In a blind funk by now I fell into the car and desperately set off again. I honestly thought I was having a heart attack and was going to die on that fateful afternoon in the Creuse. I am ashamed to admit my only thought was not of God, but hell, I didn't want to die alone in a foreign country.

Somehow I staggered into Argentan-sur-Creuse, a name now indelibly scarred onto my memory. After further palpitating moments I found the doctor's surgery and in a thoroughly un-British manner jumped the queue in the crowded waiting room. My newly acquired French totally deserted me but somehow my desperation imparted itself on the receptionist because I soon found myself ushered in to see the good doctor. He quietly and efficiently examined me and assured me that I hadn't suffered a heart attack but was *'très fatigué'*. He gave me a whole pack of prescriptions and wished me *'bonne chance'*. Now is the time to publicly thank Doctor Jean-Claude Andrieu for action that was well beyond the call of duty in my supreme hour of need.

After I had collected my prescriptions from the local pharmacy I soon found myself enjoying a luxurious soaking in my bath at a local hotel and gradually everything seemed to return to normal. Then another panic. I suddenly realized I had left my handbag (oh yes, I was pretty Frenchified by now) in the pharmacy with all my money, passport and other papers. I rocketed out of the bath and dressed in record time. As soon as I arrived back at the pharmacy, the smiling pharmacist handed back the vital item. I thanked him profusely and returned to the hotel thinking perhaps the world wasn't such a bad place after all. In my hotel room I switched on the radio and automatically tuned to Radio 4. How reassuring to hear English spoken again and in such dulcet tones. I had been speaking almost exclusively in French for over a fortnight now and I was both mentally and physically exhausted.

Then to celebrate the fact I was still alive I went out for a delicious meal in a tiny restaurant round the corner from the hotel.

The next day after my little setback in Argentan I set out refreshed and optimistic again. However the mind plays funny games with you and by lunchtime psychosomatica had taken over so I was forced to stop in that fine cathedral city of Blois straddling the Loire once again and take one of my Xanax 'Panic Pills', on which I was to rely on for so long. Xanax tablets contain the active ingredient alprazolam, which is a type of medicine called a benzodiazepine, as is diazepam, and are used as a treatment for severe anxiety, including anxiety associated with depression. They are also apparently highly addictive and only normally suitable for short-term use. They were also supposed to have the side effect of making one very drowsy. However I was to use them on and off for the next seven years with no apparent ill effects. From Blois I limped into Normandy within easy reach of Caen for the next day's crossing. On the ferry over I tried to make some sense of what had happened, and eventually decided to go and see my own doctor when I got back to England. She commenced with a structural survey and assured me that all my physical parts were in good working order. But then she delved into my mind which was a much tougher proposition altogether. She asked me if I had ever contemplated suicide and at that stage I could truthfully answer no. Then she got on to marriage and sex and I really began to squirm. I managed to divert the subject back on how to deal with my panic attacks which she had by now diagnosed as hyperventilation, and she explained the basis of correct breathing and breathing into a paper bag to help. However time was running out and she had to release me prematurely from her tender care. She had been absolutely brilliant and was just getting to the bottom of all my problems by the time the hour glass ran out.

Later the same day I abandoned my desultory attempts at packing and took to my bed again. In retrospect I just didn't realize what was happening at the time and naturally Mandy was mad at me at my 'laziness' for what was of course all my own project. She had gone along with all my great idea, however deluded, and totally despaired at my pathetic state. Of course I now realize I was in dire need of psychiatric help. After the good doctor saw me for the last time, I must have subconsciously registered that I was all alone again and slumped into a deep depression, something that had been dormant for many years. Not an ideal state of affairs.

Somehow we managed to finalize formalities and the whole family, plus aging black and tan cocker spaniel dog William, set forth for our new life appropriately enough on April Fools Day 1989, ironically also my father's birthday. Was I ready for the fray? Was I hell? It was akin to playing regularly for Sudbury Second XV and then being called up to face the might of the All Blacks at Twickenham. Oh well, *on verra*. Here we go.

Chapter 2 - Auberge Saint Martin

It was an inauspicious start to the great adventure to be heading for Dover via Norfolk that evening with my brother-in-law at the wheel. Mandy had only gone and left her passport in our desk which was at that moment at the bottom of the removal lorry in the small market town of Aylesham. Was this her subconscious telling her something? If so, we all missed it and in any event, it was too late to turn back now. By some miracle Tim, the ambidextrous removal man, managed to put a telescopic hand down, open the drawer and extract the vital document. Thus what was going to be a gentle taxi service for John became a fierce race against time. But he didn't panic, even when confronted with a late night bottleneck on the M2, and eventually deposited our motley crew at Dover Docks with a good seven minutes to spare.

Two and a half hours later we were walking through customs at Calais with William at the head and straight on to the connecting Paris train. We arrived at the Gare du Nord in Paris at about six in the morning. It was a gloriously sunny spring morning but unfortunately Daughter Number 1 got sunburnt after a trip through the Tuileries and a stroll on the Rive Gauche. The weather then declined drastically and we were hit by both hail and then a violent thunderstorm as we scrambled for the haven of the Gare du Austerlitz, an ominous shade of things to come. After a couple of hours hanging around we boarded the train again bound for our final destination, Montauban, back in the Tarn and Garonne department. We arrived at the latter station at some unholy hour where we were relieved to be met by the ever reliable Peter Davenport, a local builder, who with his wife Bernadette were always very kind to us. Peter had already created a serviceable cloakroom out of the bizarre downstairs WC behind a curtain under the stairs. On this subject the French can never understand the English obsession with multiple toilets whilst we in turn have never got to grips as it were with the ubiquitous bidet. The next day we picked up our wheels, a crappy old Talbot Horizon which we had been conned into buying from Shirley's neighbour. It did have electric windows but only half an engine and a huge dent down the side. Well, I should have remembered the old surveyors motto of caveat emptor, shouldn't I? As for buying a car unseen and without a full structural survey, that was beyond the pale. However it did get us back to Saint Martin without mishap in time for the arrival of Tim's lorry. This was of course the first time that Mandy and the girls had seen the house but I can't recall asking any of them if they approved of their new home when we arrived.

It was whilst we were waiting for Tim that I first appreciated that the elevated position of the property also gave us a disquieting early warning of the squally showers scudding at us from the south west where all the dirty weather originated from. Then Tim arrived and with his help we unloaded the lorry and the house begun to look lived in. Now we just had the simple task of converting it into an auberge.

The first task was to create another guest shower room and toilet from the front part of the large upstairs hall. Correction, the first requirement was to find the money to pay for it. I therefore flogged off the bottom field of about three hectares to another neighbour, Monsieur Sanchez, who owned the farm below us in conjunction with his father-in-law Monsieur Constantini. I have already mentioned that there were a large number of *pieds noirs* from Algeria in the region. However these 'black feet' were of very diverse origins and by 1917 it was estimated that only one European in five was of true French descent, the remainder being constituted of a very large percentage of Spanish and Italians. There are several schools of thought as to the origin of the term *pied noir*. One theory is based on the somewhat patronising view of metropolitan Frenchmen that the *colons* (European settlers) had their feet burned black by an excess of the African sun. Another one that appeals to me referred to sailors working in the coal room of a steam ship. For these bare-footed workers, having feet blackened by the coal and sun was an occupational hazard. In the Mediterranean, the coal room worker was more often than not an Algerian, and so the term evolved from being a derogatory term for an Algerian, to being used to a person of French descent born in Algeria. A third more prosaic theory is based on account of the fact that the French military wore black polished shoes.

In the event I only got forty thousand francs for my land from my wily neighbour, not fifty as promised by Max Miquel. However after a swift sale of the land I got another rude shock when I discovered that although the purchaser obviously has to pay over all the money when signing the *acte,* not so obviously the seller doesn't correspondingly receive the money straightaway. The reason proved to be entirely logical as ever, if infinitely frustrating. The *notaire* has to check with the *Bureau de Hypothèques* that between the *Sous-Seeing* and the *Acte* the seller hasn't pulled a fast one by taking out a mortgage on the property and nipped off with the proceeds. The idea is OK in principle but one is totally in the hands of bureaucratic delay. In the event the money came through in the nick of time to pay Monsieur Vanzetti for the excellent work he had done on the shower room. Monsieur Bergmans, an eccentric but wildly enthusiastic Belgian, was also to prove an able plumber with the incongruous assistance of his plumber's mate, his rather large daughter. His finished product was highly efficient but more in the style of Richard Rogers Pompidou Centre with all the pipes hanging out. Our electrics were also rather dodgy with some worrying scorch marks around a number of plugs. Monsieur Rouilles was in charge here and did a great job on the safety front. English immigrant electricians were always quick to criticize the French ringmayne system with its apparent lack of earthing but the only fire I came across in my seven years in France was caused by an electrical fault where the work was carried out by an Englishman. Enough said.

We were gradually getting there and next we called in Cézanne to do the painting (i.e. yours truly). I was of course very much a brains not brawn man but this was to be one of my finest hours. We had five bedrooms, a large hall and two bathrooms upstairs to do plus substantial sundries on the ground floor. As the ceilings were over three metres high, the task was both intimidating and fraught with danger, although I found the tie bars useful in this respect for hanging onto. Anyway I completed the task unscathed but sweating profusely in the searing heat as summer had arrived promptly on May 1st.

Then I returned to see the mediaeval mayor's secretary, this time armed with all the necessary documentation, together with the rest of the family. We drove up a rutted stone path to the loud barking of assorted canines. The old two storey farmhouse was of stone also, looking worn away around its edges as it balanced over a steep precipice. An old couple peered out suspiciously at our young family who had turned up unannounced at their private fiefdom. However they eventually realized we were not dangerous and had simply come on the mayor's business. We were ushered in out of the bright sunlight into the mayor's secretary '*bureau*' which appeared to be the main living room of the house to the right of the front door. With the shutters firmly shut against the heat, the room appeared to be in almost total darkness. However the secretary merely put on a tiny pair of reading glasses and appeared to have adapted totally to the gloom. As he rummaged away in his desk for the appropriate forms, our eyes slowly adjusted to the light, or rather to the lack of it. The room appeared to be like the inside of a bric-a-brac shop with heavy old furniture filling it to the gunnels and littered with all manner of papers. Eventually even the secretary deemed it necessary for us to have some sort of illumination so that we could participate in this bit of officialdom. He reached a brown sinewy hand up to a tiny cord hanging from what I assumed to be an ornamental antique lamp. The latter flickered intermittently into life but instead of throwing some light on the proceedings, merely gave out a fading yellowy glow that added only shadows. In spite of all his pernicketyness, the old secretary was most efficient and very precise, even if it felt at the time like we were partaking in some Dickensian melodrama. We were soon blinking our way out back into the brilliant sunlight with all necessary forms duly signed and stamped. The Turner family had arrived: nos. 307-311 of the population of the commune of Mauroux.

In the meantime the girls had their first day of French school at the little village of Marsac about five kilometers away. Unfortunately it was across the border back in the Tarn and Garonne and this created the usual logistical and administrative problems. Roger had recommended it and again he came up trumps. The petite and charming Madame Rodrigues was the *directrice* aided and abetted by two enthusiastic and talented *professeurs*. All the girls' future success was down to those vital formative years. However I still remember vividly that first morning dropping the girls off and saw them all troop in forlornly. Daughter Number 1 was eight years old, Daughter Number 2 six and Daughter Number 3 only four. It was a poignant moment and I thought morosely what on earth had I let them into? I am now so proud of all they have achieved since that grey April day in 1989. The junior school had fifty *élèves* from ten years old all the way down to two. The French system overall is chronically over structured but it certainly served our girls well, especially when they returned to face the English curriculum and its loose, undisciplined ways.

Back on the auberge front I had managed to wangle a hundred thousand pound loan from the friendly director of the local Crédit Agricole bank in Saint Clar. The latter was a classical *bastide* (fortified small town) dating back to the thirteenth century and co-founded by Edward 1st of England. Indeed English influence was everywhere with it all originating from Eleanor of Aquitaine in 1153 when she married Henry Plantagenet, Duke of Anjou, who was soon to be crowned Henry the Second of England. Eleanor and Henry were also the main players in that fine sixties film, The Lion in Winter, starring Katherine Hepburn, Peter O'Toole and a very youthful Anthony Hopkins in his first film. Unfortunately it all ended in tears and a lot of dead bodies with The Hundred Years War. I discovered from Roger that Saint Martin had once had its own commune with over five hundred inhabitants, but most of the men folk had been killed in that terrible *hécatombe* (slaughter) and Saint Martin had subsequently been absorbed by Mauroux. The hamlet now had only six surviving habitable properties, including a chateau co-owned by three Dutch families, but there was only one other house permanently occupied apart from ours. Saint Clar had a typically Gascon *place* with stone archways all round where the summer garlic festival was held. Saint Clar was the joint garlic (*ail*) capital of France together with Beaumont de Lomagne. The indigenous limestone of the Lomagne region was also a notable building feature and Saint Clar was a fine example of its use. Only around half of the properties in the village were occupied, a sad pattern repeated in nearly all the nearby villages. The Gers was the most agricultural department in the country and only had a population of one hundred and eighty thousand inhabitants. The area had originally been mostly pasture and woodland but the arrival of the subsidized irrigation lakes in the early Sixties had transformed the landscape into a kind of overheated East Anglian wasteland. Oh yes, it didn't take me long to become a French NIMBY. Six months earlier I had never heard of the Gers but I was already pontificating to them on the error of their ways. On a more serious note the rural population was being continuously eroded by the drift to the towns and cities because the sons of small arable farmers were deserting the countryside in droves. Hence the acquiescence and even approval of the local inhabitants of the sudden invasion by *les rosbifs* (this time peaceful with credit card in hand rather than pitchfork and longbow) buying up unwanted ruins with the huge benefits to local shopkeepers and builders, even if they were somewhat mystified by it all. Try to imagine a reciprocal Gallic invasion of Suffolk. You can't, can you? Much later I was asked directly about this phenomenon by a friend at the local golf club and had to admit the main reason for buying was the incredibly cheap property prices, followed by the incredibly cheap property prices and then finally by the incredibly cheap property prices. Qualities such as the ambience, wide open places, climate and beautiful countryside followed at a very respectful distance.

Where was I? Oh yes, trying to make a living. I should have listened to that wise old farmer who after I had waxed lyrical about his marvellous location, simply said 'bugger the views, they don't pay the bills'. Profound words that I should have listened more carefully to at the time and which were to come back and haunt me later. *Enfin* by July we were ready to repel boarders and had a little party to celebrate and to thank all the locals who had helped us to fulfil our dreams, or should I say my dream. It was a lovely summer's evening and as we were regaled by a glorious sunset from the terrace I reflected not that it had been mad to come but that it would have been *fou (mad)* not to. My property problems seemed a million miles away and David Soul's winsome Silver Lady suddenly sprung to mind.

'Tired of drifting, searching, shifting through town to town
Every time I slip and slide a little bit further down
I can't blame you if you won't take me back
After everything I put you through
But honey you're my last hope
And who else can I turn to.

Come on Silver Lady take my word
I won't run out on you again believe me
Oh, I've seen the light
It's just one more fight
Without you
Here I am a million miles from home
The Indiana wind and rain cut through me
I'm lost and alone, chilled to the bone
Silver Lady.'

Totally inappropriate words for a Gascon summer I know, but perhaps I was just subconsciously registering that Saint Martin itself was 'my last hope', if not Mandy herself. *Aucune idée* (no idea).

I also heard from Shirley's husband that England had been thrashed by Australia in the first Ashes Test Match and didn't even care. Blimey, I must have been getting seriously Frenchifried already. Or perhaps, more insidiously, it showed the magnitude of my escape from reality.

Our first clients were a charming young Dutch couple and it felt good to receive my first bit of income in almost nine months. However they also unwittingly graphically illustrated two major problems. First they were chain smokers and we were immediately worried by the fire hazard in the bedrooms. Of course in those good old days the banning of smoking in public places was but a gleam in the eye of the health police. At this stage I would also like to stick my neck out once again by stating that the Dutch are the heaviest smokers in northern Europe and the meanest tippers. Scotsmen and Yorkshiremen seem positively profligate in comparison. Those statements are not meant to be unkind. Our Dutch neighbours were all delightful and often brilliant linguists, although one could again uncharitably argue that with such an ugly language they needed to be. 'To be fair' it has to be said that a large number of Brits couldn't help being a pain abroad, even more so than at home. With their incredibly poor dress sense, burnt skin and loud Anglo Saxon voices, they were a constant embarrassment in bars, supermarkets and on the beaches. Thank God we had all returned home by the time that the lager louts invaded Toulouse during the World Cup in 1998. And to borrow from Professor Higgins *un petit peu*, why can't the English teach their children how to speak foreign languages?

The other rather delicate problem arising from the Dutch couple's sojourn was soundproofing, or rather the lack of it. We had these unplastered ceilings on the ground floor which, whilst they exposed the fine timber beams to perfection, they also graphically exposed normal nocturnal activity. What to do? Nothing, except to turn a discreet Nelson's ear and hope other guests weren't in the firing line so to speak at an inopportune moment. Of course this is another Anglo Saxon *faiblesse*. Other less sexually oppressed repressed nations literally couldn't care a fuck. On reading this paragraph my wife has made the unhelpful suggestion that Englishman may specialize in the stiff upper lip, that is about the only item of their anatomy which remains in that state. Who am I to argue? Roll on Viagra on the National Health.

Back on the business front we had received our precious *Carte de Séjour* with the benevolent assistance of Monsieur Dubarry and also obtained the official Licence for the auberge from the Chamber of Commerce at Auch, the departmental capital of the Gers and some forty five kilometers to the south. Auch itself is a delightful small town with a fine cathedral and very strong connections with D'Artagnan from Dumas, who of course needs no introducing. Anyone who has been up all one hundred steps to see his statue has certainly earned his *pastis*. Auch is also one of the most unpronounceable names of all French towns. If you haven't already been let into the secret don't try it, although an Anglicized *Orsh* wouldn't be too far away.

By getting registered into the official French system we were now entitled to the substantial child benefit of over two thousand francs a month, but this was more than nullified by our *Cotizations* or compulsory private schemes for pensions, illness and unemployment benefits. These needed to be paid up front with large minimum subscriptions, even if you weren't trading at a profit. Somehow we managed to avoid the onerous fire precautions or a drinks licence because at that stage we were only trading as a bed and breakfast establishment.

We had advertised in English publications like the Lady, Country Life and The Independent newspaper as we were of course far too late to get into any travel guide.   I was working very much on an ad hoc basis with no master plan, business plan or in fact any plan at all. The so called business loan had already been extravagantly swallowed up on essential items and not so essential frivolities. On the booking side we had been greatly aided by an article I wrote for The Independent which I publish below with their kind permission, together with their amusing and darkly ironic cartoon.

DEPARTURES

Cautionary tale for enterprising readers

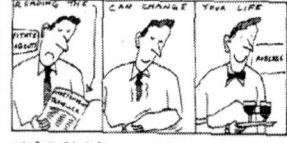

PERHAPS the *Independent Traveller* ought to carry some sort of warning: "Reading this section can change your life." It certainly did for Simon Turner, who read a feature on these pages a year ago written by Godfrey Hodgson on his travels around the Michelin "Red Rocker" hotels in the region around Toulouse in south-west France.

Mr Turner was a chartered surveyor who worked for Hampton's estate agents, but had realised that he "patiently wasn't" suited to selling houses". He confessed that at the age of 40 he had reached "the proverbial midlife crisis" and was searching for a different way of life.

"I had holidayed several times in France and was toying with the idea of buying a house there, but with no definite plan in mind. I had already received details of properties in several regions of France, including the Toulouse area, when I providentially read your article, 'At the sign of the Red Rocker', the catalyst being the mention of a cheap flight to Toulouse from Heathrow for £114 return."

He immediately booked a flight to Toulouse, saw a house 35 miles north-west of Toulouse in a small hamlet and realised it was ideal as a home as well as an auberge. "I discussed the matter with my wife and signed a contract straight away — without my wife seeing the house, I then left Hampton's and spent two months at the Berlitz School of Language in London."

Mr Turner his wife and three daughters aged eight, six and four moved to France in April and his auberge opened in July. The three children are now attending the local village school. "Despite various teething problems we are very happy in our new life," said Mr Turner.

"The auberge is an attractive nineteenth-century house standing in a secluded garden of about one acre with glorious views towards the Pyrenees. Guests have the use of the spacious ground-floor living room with direct access to the large south-facing terrace. There are also swings and a games room for the children." There are three rooms available; one double, one single and a family room.

Bed and breakfast prices are around £10 per person for adults, £5 for children (aged four to 12), children under four are free. Evening meals on request at £8 per person. Mid-life crisis readers are duly warned.

Simon and Mandy Turner, Saint-Martin, Mauroux, 32380 Saint-Clar (010 33 62 66 49 32).

We had three letting bedrooms that first summer and made the first of numerous errors by grossly undercharging; a hundred and fifty francs only fully inclusive bed and board with a four course evening meal thrown in together with house wine and coffee. Derisory. For breakfast I always nipped in for fresh croissants and baguettes, plus the local *La Dépêche* (despatch) newspaper and the previous day's Times, a good catholic mélange. Sophie and her husband made the best bread in the Lomagne, their specialties being *tournesol, orge* and *blé* (sunflowers, barley and wheat respectively). Tragically they were both killed five years later in a motor cycle accident.

Our first block of guests were all very pleasant and included a journalist and his wife, another couple and a very quiet gentleman who we discovered had just lost his wife to the dreadful wasting motor neurone disease.

Christ, it was hot. The hottest time of day in this part of the world proved not be lunchtime as in England but around four o'clock, although even at eight in the evening it was still too hot for most people on the south facing terrace. It was then that we discovered the true value of shutters as they created an oasis of cool and darkness in the house compared to the searing heat outside.

Mandy did all the cooking and hard sweat whilst I was the genial host dispensing drinks and urbanity in equal measure. Unfortunately later on some hardline Thatcherites really got up my nose and I deteriorated into a poor man's Basil Fawlty. The girls were put to work and soon became proficient and charming *serveuses,* even if I say so myself, and backed up with some very generous *pourboires* or tips. My pride and joy was the tiled floor which stretched over the whole of the vast open plan ground floor. I cosseted and polished it to an incredible sheen and even admonished guests who marked it with their trainers. People who know me now may find that a trifle hard to believe but it was a true reflection of my increasingly obsessive behaviour. My other obsession was the cow pasture of a garden which extended to about an acre, where I sweated blood liberally and literally when the vicious horseflies descended on my unprotected back. After a couple of months I had tamed the wilderness and was tolerably proud of my efforts. The following year it almost broke my heart when the *pelle mécanique* (JCB) gouged out a great gash in it to prepare for the new *fosse septique* (septic tank). In this respect I must mention in despatches Michel, the master machine operator, who was so expert at his job that he could caress a beer bottle top off with his JCB.

On the construction front we also had delivered lorry loads of gravel at the front where I redid the drive and also created a high class *pétanque* area. I had one of the most satisfying days of my life trundling up and down on the mini steam roller I had hired to finish the job off. Yes, back to my school days where I could just be a little boy again and not have to face up to real life. By now the auberge was quite transformed from the dark and dingy property I had acquired only three months earlier. Our neighbours were brilliant except for the randy Monsieur Fignon who luckily only descended from Bordeaux for the long summer holidays. Monsieur Magnier was great if you could understand any of his guttural patois but we gathered he was especially pleased that we had brought a young family with us to live there all year round. Monsieur and Madame Duvasse were the local *foie gras* experts and for all those rabid animal righters who were vocally opposed to *le gavage* (stuffing or alleged force feeding of geese and ducks) I can assure you it is impossible to operate this system on an unhappy bird. In fact the geese and ducks spent the vast majority of their lives in excellent free range conditions, in marked contrast to the vast majority of their British counterparts. It was only at the very end of their lives that *le gavage* was applied to them. More on *le gavage* later.

On the auberge front everything went swimmingly (an extremely unfortunate phrase as you will soon discover) until my sister and the rest of her family arrived one blistering August afternoon. After tea and all the pleasantries had been concluded it was time for drinkies and the mighty Baron, a five franc sparkly we had discovered in Brittany about five years earlier. It was always guaranteed to improve the spirits whatever the mood, which was just as well on account of the events to be unfurled. We had desultorily noticed the skies clouding over but thought nothing of it. Then they went an eerie pink and everything was ominously still. We still weren't too fussed as the Baron continued to flow liberally. Suddenly, without any warning at all, it happened. First a hurricane like wind arose from nowhere and then the thunderstorm hit us amidships. A month earlier we had enjoyed a pyrotechnic extravaganza of forked lightning from afar, but this time we were the entertainment. The wind was so strong we could barely secure the shutters, but our respite was short lived because the next thing we knew we had water pouring into the lounge living area from above. Thoroughly alarmed I went to investigate upstairs and was horrified by what I found. In one of the front bedrooms part of the ceiling had been sucked up by the storm. Even worse was to come when we went up to the *grenier* (attic) and found that the wind had lifted the unsecured tiles up at right angles and the rain was just pouring through the gaping holes. I summoned by brother-in-law to the rescue. First he smashed back the escaping ceiling and then made further use of his Joel Garner reach by forcing the errant tiles back one by one. John certainly earned his Saint Martin cap that evening. As suddenly as it arose the storm abated and I was quite reasonably left to do all the mopping up after my meagre contribution. The incident left me seriously shaken and stirred and whenever storm clouds gathered around the not so magic hour of seven o'clock in the evening in the future I was always a nervous wreck.

We had been very lucky with all our guests up to now but I sensed seeds of trouble with the coming of the formidable Mrs Randall and her husband in early September. But *attention*, appearances can be deceptive. The second afternoon she marched into our private kitchen without knocking and I thought what the hell's gone wrong now? However she had only come in to bring the children some delicious patisserie. Gwen and Stan only stayed a week but in all our time in France they never failed to send a bumper parcel to the girls for Christmas. What a generous couple.

Towards the end of our first season we certainly hadn't made any money but were very pleased with progress in general. The girls had settled in brilliantly at school even if their French was inevitably struggling. They also thoroughly appreciated the ten week *grandes vacances*. However it was tough for Mandy in the broiler house of a kitchen but she created some marvellous meals and coped with the radical change of scene stoically. One of our last guests of the year in late November was PSJ and his partner Wendy. He was sniffing round for a little ruin so I put him in touch with Shirley and she soon found him a nice little country property near the girls' school at Marsac. Oh and that reminds me Shirley, I am still waiting ever so patiently for my promised introductory fee. No hurry.

Despite our very modest success in our first year I realized we had to maximize the cashflow situation by somehow elongating it over a full twelve months rather than just a four month summer season. The trouble was that, contrary to popular conception, the climate in the Gers wasn't consistently sunny and mild all the year round like on the Riviera to the east. The Victorians certainly knew a thing or two about holidays. The summers were certainly very hot but there were frequent thunderstorms as well as incredible changes in temperature. In fact the only thing consistent about the weather was its inconsistency. One year it rained every day in May, another every day in October, while once we even had a week's freezing fog when my parents were staying and the frost froze all the telephone wires white.

Back to cashflow. Mandy's cooking had proved very popular and we decided to open a restaurant to the general public in the New Year. I spent fifteen thousand francs on *panneaux* or advertising boards all over the place, no planning permission needed only owner's permission, and then sat back and waited for business to flood in. The trouble was that I hadn't done my sums again. If I had just sat down and done the maths, I would have realized it was impossible to get my money back on the signs, however popular the restaurant might prove to be, due to the lack of covers. The numbers just didn't add up. Another fifteen hundred quid down the drain. The main problem was that old location, location location mantra. Saint Martin was literally in the middle of nowhere which, while great for a quiet holiday, wasn't so good when you were trying to make some money. Again a teeny weeny bit of business nous would have told me that in the first place, but I still 'didn't get it', to utilize another topical catch phrase. Nevertheless, as the weather warmed up in the New Year business began to pick up promisingly, although the ultra conservative locals took a hell of a lot of persuading. And the pressure. I don't know how top chefs do it year on year. With the Chambre d'Hôte you had the chance up to a week or more to cultivate the clients, but with the restaurant it was a strictly one off affair with no second chance. Although we always tried to encourage people to book in advance if possible, there were always clients coming off the streets as it were. We got a very early break when three satisfied lunchtime customers announced that they were from the Guide Gascon and that we would be in it the following season. On their next visit the following season Mandy was back in England for one of her nieces' confirmation and so I was left in charge to hold the fort. I managed to do enough to persuade the selectors to retain our place in the Guide for the following year. We also hosted a large gathering of the local *Chambre d'Agriculteurs* which was another feather in our cap as well as useful money in the bank. At this moment I crave a spot of indulgence by letting the Guide Gascon of 1991/2 wax lyrical on our behalf:-

'Nos amis Anglais reviennent dans une region que leurs ancètres connaissent bien : la Gascogne.

Cette maison de pierre vient d'être transformée par Mandy and Simon Turner en auberge. Nous avons apprécié, non seulement la cuisine ou la touche anglaise est perceptible, mais aussi la discrétion de la famille Turner. Le couvert est raffiné, les plats très bien présentés et vous serez servis a table par Simon Turner et l'une des trois filles de la maison. Tres beau panorama: Saint Martin est un des points culminants du département.'

Pas mal, hein?

Drinks were supplied courtesy of Monsieur Matuzzio and there were a number of excellent local wines, the best being the fruity Côtes de Saint Mont white, the ruby red Buzet and the gutsy Madiran, pearl of the reds. Pelforth Blond was the preferred beer, whilst the Pelforth Brune made a surprisingly good stout in winter. However the summer temperatures were too hot for dehydrating beers, which is why the locals drink pastis with plenty of water. And last but not least came 'That Naughty Floc', as Gwen Randall quaintly christened it, or more formally Floc de Gascogne, a delicious fortified sweet wine with both red and white varieties.

By this time William had suffered from more and more infirmities and one morning he just looked at me beseechingly. He had just had enough. Later in the day I took him to a sympathetic vet at Lectoure where he was quietly put down. We had been through a lot together. We had acquired him in Cape Town and then he had to suffer the inhumanity of six months quarantine when we returned to England. He then had eleven good years there before ending his days in France. Not a bad dog's life.

It is always very sad losing an old friend and we vowed never to have another dog. However fate was to prove otherwise. The following Christmas we made the long trip back to England to see all the family. Just before we left a middle-aged beagle hound turned up on our doorstep unannounced. We kept her for a few days but no one came to claim her and she was still there on the doorstep when we returned from our week in England. Of course we had to keep her and christened her Peggy. However I must say here and now that Peggy proved to be the most deceitful and promiscuous beagle in the Gers. Before Christmas she had been as good as gold but once she realized we had taken her in she reverted to all her old obviously well engrained bad habits. She took off hunting for up to three days at a time whenever she felt like it and came back exhausted and with scratches all over her body. She quickly became pregnant (father unknown) and in time she had her first motley litter with us, although I strongly suspect that she wasn't a virgin when she first ingratiated herself on us. Later she had sex with one of her own sons in full view of the children and carried on her thoroughly delinquent ways to the end of her days. However for some unfathomable reason Mandy seemed to prefer her to me.

On to more edifying subjects. We had a steady stream of clients in the early months of 1990 for the auberge including Marion Kaplan and Eric Robbins, both expats from Portugal who were to become regular visitors. They were both writers and gave first Mandy, and very belatedly myself, the inspiration to take up the pen. We also had our first Germans and I found it bloody difficult not to talk about the war. We also had a good percentage of Dutch customers and a fair sprinkling of French. Then in early May we had another couple back who were going to do something similar to us back in Beaumont. On their first evening they had just finished drinks on the terrace and casually remarked that the weather looked a bit threatening. Quarter of an hour later they had just embarked on their soup when another storm struck. Literally five minutes after that water was pouring into the dining area through the floor boards above and I was soon mopping up a lake. But the British are not anything if resourceful and we completed the meal as the storm raged. Neither were our phlegmatic diners phased at all. In fact later they remarked that they hadn't had as much fun for years and it also gave them a story to dine out to for years to come. An hour later you wouldn't have known that anything had happened at all downstairs. Upstairs it was a different story as the whitewashed walls were now colour washed and we eventually got the insurance company to pay out for the large repainting job.

We also had some regular business from the nearby nudist colony. I had to visit the site once (I can't think on what pretext) and took the girls along. Having seen a string of bulging bottoms and assorted shrivelled tits and willies, Daughter No 2 came out with the obvious comment 'they're all bare'. Of course they were and there were also the odd splendid bronzed titties and whatnots (let's not beat about the bush) to satisfy the most ardent voyeur.

However other types of storm clouds were gathering on the horizon, namely financial ones. I had long used up our bank facility but Dad provided more funds which managed both to keep the Crédit Agricole at bay for the moment and to finance the hire purchase of a new car, namely a Volkswagen Golf. This car proved to be very faithful and not only took us through to the end of our stay in France, but lasted another ten years back in England into the bargain. The French had a very good system of charging Road Fund Tax in different bands according to the age, value and size of engine of the car. Therefore if you had an old banger like the Horizon you only paid four hundred and fifty francs, while a new Roller would cost you the maximum of eight thousand francs. At the same time as we bought the Golf I had to pay to have the old Horizon towed away. Typical of my poor timing, the next year the government brought in an incentive to buy new cars by providing five thousand francs for any old banger, which our government copied almost twenty years later and the Golf missed reaching by a similar twelve months. *C'est la vie.*

Of course it didn't take much financial acumen to work out that we would never have made nearly enough profit from the auberge to provide even an adequate family income. But of course my financial brain still wasn't working. Dad wanted to help but it was probably the worst move he could have made to bail me out again and keep a sinking ship away from the rocks for another tantalizing period.

During all this time we had been remarkably lucky with guests and diners alike. However the non-human elements continued to give us grief. Unusually I was resting on my laurels on the terrace one sultry afternoon underneath the shade of the rapacious Russian vine when I heard a loud rustling immediately above me. I glanced up and saw an enormous green and yellow snake. Roger scornfully informed me later that it was just a *coulèvre* (grass snake) *'pas méchant'* but I was not totally convinced and that *endroit* had totally lost its charm after that incident. Later on I was also discouraged from spending much time in the rough on the golf course when I came across one of those horrible vipers. It wasn't all fun and games in the Gers. We were then inundated for a short period by the ominous zzzz of massive frélons (hornets). My brother-in-law again came into to his own on another flying visit. We always put him to work when he came. The hornets used to rest on the beams and again he used his great height to great effect by swatting them like flies. I had to stand on a chair to reach them and the blighters usually nipped off before I could wield a heavy hand or glove. They were far worse at night as they were attracted in by the lights. On one occasion one of my French guests ignored our warning and left the windows of his bedroom open with the result that there about half a dozen of the buggers swarming round the main light. To the encouraging shouts of *'bravo monsieur'* I swatted the lot with the assistance of Country Life or some such pornographic material. After that we managed to trace the nest and the very efficient *pompiers* (firemen) did the rest.

Come the New Year the financial situation was really grave again so naturally I took to my bed with increasing regularity. Mandy was beside herself in a strange country with little French (oh yes I had seen to that since I hardly let her out and did all the external negotiations myself) and no near family or close friends but I was oblivious. My mental condition wasn't exactly ameliorated by another crippling panic attack when the family were out of the house for a couple of hours. This time I just lay on my bed and sweated profusely and with wild palpitations my heart felt it was going to explode. Eventually with the help of my old Xanax 'Panic Pills' again the symptoms subsided and I realized not exactly with relief that I was still alive. Naturally I didn't mention the episode to Mandy on her return.

Miraculously the children seemed to be relatively unscathed by it all and suddenly we realized they were speaking amongst themselves in French, a habit they have continued to this day. Contrary to popular opinion all kids don't learn a new language effortlessly and quickly and it took the girls a full eighteen months before they became completely fluent. They had all acquired Gascon accents with Daughter No 3's being the most authentic of all, which was not surprising as she first learned both to read and write in French. Luckily they were still too young to realize the financial problems even if they were aware that Daddy 'wasn't very well'. Eventually I swung back into something like sanity as the new season got under way, but my heart was no longer in it and I found myself arguing vociferously with Tory ladies about the iniquity of the Poll Tax.

Up to now we had still been remarkably lucky with all our guests. Therefore when a rather odd character turned up late in the evening just before dinner, I didn't pay him much attention though he appeared to be sweating excessively even allowing for the heat. We had fourteen for dinner that evening including several old friends. Suddenly after supper we realized that he seemed to have disappeared and were panic struck when we realized that Daughter No 3 wasn't with the other two girls as we thought. Up to now one of the great charms of the place was that it was such a safe and peaceful place to bring up the children. With the other guests we carried out an increasingly desperate search. Just when we had reached the end of our tether, with a mixture of elation and horror we saw her returning hand in hand with our strange visitor. As he vehemently denied anything had happened we could only belatedly warn him to keep away from the children. He took the hint and retired to bed. However I still couldn't relax and stayed up all night to ensure there were no further incidents. The weirdo left rapidly in the morning but not before I had taken his car registration number and phoned the local gendarmerie. After that unfortunate incident what little was left of my heart went out of my dream project and I proceeded to vet potential clients as closely as they inspected their rooms. I managed to really upset one very posh French lady by turning away her and her two little dogs despite my eminently reasonable explanation that Peggy was on heat (*en chaleur*) again and we had quite enough little Peggys already thank you very much. Naturally this didn't go down very well and a couple of weeks later I received a fierce diatribe not exactly extolling my virtues.

Things couldn't get any worse, could they? Early in August a sprightly septuagenarian widow arrived with her daughter. After a splendid evening they set out in great heart the next morning on their hire bikes. In the afternoon while I was hiding from the world upstairs in our bedroom Mandy received a call from the daughter to say that her mother had been hit by a motorbike and was in intensive care in Auch hospital. In quick succession the rest of the family arrived and she was eventually taken off by air ambulance to England where she fortunately recovered.

However don't go away with the idea that it was all doom and gloom. One of our very last group of guests was an interesting threesome, one lady and two men. The former was obviously very pious because she carefully asked for the exact time and place for Mass the next morning. She was chaperoned by her brother and her builder, the latter being a six foot six coloured gentleman of few words, and they carefully booked into three separate rooms. However when I knocked on her door in the morning to wake her for Mass, although the voice that answered appeared to be feminine the snoring was indubitably masculine. Later when Mandy was cleaning out her room she informed me that she had found some quick release knickers, whatever they might be, under the pillow. I couldn't care a toss what consenting adults got up to in private but why the hypocrisy and the expense of an extra room?

On that inappropriate bonking note we wound up Auberge Saint Martin at Christmas, an inglorious and inevitable failure.

Chapter 3 - Agent Immobilier

One spring morning in 1991 I woke for once with a clear head and employed a little bit of that fossilized grey matter that had been decaying quietly for some time. It was blindingly obvious. I would return to property, the only occupation I knew anything about. And as Johnny Nash sung so cheerfully all those years ago:-

'I can see clearly now, the rain is gone,
I can see all the obstacles in my way
Gone are the dark clouds that had me blind
It's gonna be a bright (bright) bright (bright)
Sun-shiny day.'

But was Johnny right?

I had just about recovered from the Hamptons sacking (had I hell) and the only other obstacle had been a misguided loyalty to Shirley Temple. However after the latter had reneged on her dues over PSJ's purchase, I now had no compunction at being in direct competition with her. Not that she would have noticed anyway. My next obstacle was to find who to join and that was the start of another difficulty. In France the whole estate agency business was totally different to that prevailing in England. In England any Tom, Dick or Colonel Ponsonby can setup overnight with zero capital and zero expertise. What a crappy system. Of course there the mighty Royal Institution of Chartered Surveyors or the mini M.N.A.E. but they are only advisory, not compulsory bodies. In England we seem to be slaves to self-regulation, a policy that has recently come back to haunt the country with the recent banking crisis, to say nothing of Members of Parliament expenses. In France they go to the other extreme. Every *agence immobilier* must hold the all important '*carte professionelle' (Loi Hoguet)*. In order to obtain this vital scrap of paper you had to meet specific legal academic conditions. The theory was excellent but seriously flawed in practice for two main reasons. First of all the people with the vital card before the relevant date (20/7/72) were often only insurance agents with no expertise of property at all. The second flaw was the threat to the hegemony of *notaires.* Previously the latter had both been broking the deal while at the same time advising both parties on a notionally neutral manner on legal matters. *Ce n'est pas possible, mon petit.*

Anyway my timing as ever was impeccable. After three years when any medium mature *mec* (bloke) could have sold French ruins to naive British buyers like myself, the bubble burst with the almost simultaneous collapse of the English economy and property market and later concomitant collapse of the pound against the franc. From a high when I bought Saint Martin two years earlier of around eleven francs to the pound, after Black Wednesday it had sunk by over twenty five per cent of its value to around eight before disappearing down the plughole at 7.33.

But I still had the problem of which agency to join. In my travels I had noticed a promising looking agency in the rugged hillside town of Lectoure and another one in the market town of Fleurance with its unsurpassed Place and Arches. In the latter town there was also the Lou Fleuret Café which served the best coffee in the Gers. At Lou's the coffee was fresh, not too bitter and of course scaldingly hot. The secret of good coffee making is like that of well kept real ale is that key is in both the coffee grains and the pipes. Of course, I was a bit of an expert in the coffee stakes, even if, like Louis XIV, I say so myself. When I've got a spare moment I might write the definitive good coffee guide to Gascony. Should be another best seller if I ever have enough energy to lift up my pen again. Sadly for true aficionados, Lou subsequently sold his business. He told me he used to sell about two hundred cups of coffee a day. It may not sound much but multiply it through at five francs a cup and you arrive at the figure of one thousand francs a day of three hundred and sixty five thousand francs a year on coffee alone. *Pas mal, hein?*

I approached a Monsieur Van Gogh at Fleurance as a first step and he seemed quite interested. He also apparently worked with Monsieur Lacapère at Lectoure so everything in the garden should have been rosy, but of course I should have been immediately suspicious of the short, fat and beady-eyed M Van Gogh who was another former insurance agent. In any event it was all very low key for a couple of months which left me plenty of time to try and prop up the Auberge. Then one day Jean-Paul, my French *confrère*, excitedly asked for my assistance with some English clients. We quickly got them interested in a dilapidated old farmhouse just outside Saint Clar. We equally quickly got them to agree the price with the vendors, unfortunately with the aggressive pressing of M. Van Gogh in attendance. The latter also miraculously produced a contract for me to sign which I did without looking at the small print, or the large print for that matter. Later this omission was to cost me very dearly. I took the prospective purchasers home to Saint Martin for tea and comfort. Eventually they seemed a bit more relaxed about the purchase until I committed a cardinal error. They were still feeling the pressure exerted by M Van Gogh and wanted some solicitors in England who specialized in French conveyancing to look at the contract. I tried to persuade them against this action so that the contract could be signed *tout de suite* in the morning. However when I phoned their chambre d'hôte the next morning I found they had done a runner. Evidently I had scared them off with my own form of pressurizing. I found out later they had bought the same property in due course from a local agent or *marchand de biens* (or licensed speculator). First client and first sale cockup, not a very promising start to my *immobilier* career.

My second clients came directly from a little ad that I had placed in the Sunday Times. They were another English family who had not only sold their property in England but also came to stay at Saint Martin with us for the weekend. A sitting duck you might have thought, or *un canard anglais*, but in both cases you would be well wrong to use the modern if ugly vernacular. In mitigation I would plead that I did find them the house of their dreams, again with the help of Jean-Paul. The property hadn't officially come onto the market yet but Jean-Paul was confident that we could manage to seal the deal this time. The house was a typical mellow stone Gascon farmhouse with about seven hectares and lovely views up the Gimone valley. It was rumoured that someone else was interested in the property but we didn't for a moment believe that old *blague* (joke, or more likely con), especially in France where property was traditionally slower to shift. I therefore left Graham, my client, to ruminate on it while he drove back to England. He then phoned me back a couple of days later and told me to go for it. Unbelievably for me the ugly rumour was true (but no, it wasn't Mr Blair). It was a local doctor who had already signed on the dotted line. Even more unbelievably it was only about eight hundred metres along the road from the other purchasers' house. Every time I drove along the D7 to Tournecoupe after that I had two jagged reminders of my failures.

Neither did it help when Graham bought his second choice straightaway from another agent as he had to complete before the *rentrée* for the children. Ironically I was to sell the charcoal remains of this property some five years later after he had retired financially hurt to England. A miraculous fire had already proved to be his financial salvation as I had negotiated a large insurance settlement for him. I wouldn't have minded a bit of his luck, especially when you bear in mind that the fire had been caused by a fault in the wiring which had been carried out by an English electrician. If I had been acting for the other side, I would have made a strong recommendation against paying out to the insurance company.

I had already had several unfruitful dealings so far with the Gersois version of Arthur Daley, a loveable rogue (*mon dieu* that sounds condescending) but with his once fine features bloated and ravaged by alcohol and tragedy. His wife, a local schoolteacher, had apparently committed suicide in particularly grisly fashion some years earlier. However he was usually a jovial, rotund figure of fun if again rather vertically challenged. He also had a heart of gold which he carefully tried to hide. He once gave me part of his own commission to give to the girls as he knew how much I was struggling to survive. On the subject of size it was strange that there seemed to be so many Gascon midgets floating about when we were in the heartland of French rugby with all those massive *piliers* (props), *talonneurs* (hookers) and *troisième lignes* (back row forwards) skulking about in the undergrowth. We were also in Condom country, a name forever associated with the orally challenged Young Nigel. For those younger readers amongst you by Young Nigel I am actually referring to the eternally puckish Nigel Starmer-Smith who was a very enthusiastic rugby commentator in the 1970's, 80's and 90's,and number two for the BBC to the late, great Bill Maclaren. Young Nigel for some reason showed great reluctance to admit that Jean Condom, that fine French second row forward, was ever actually on the field of combat despite the fact that he played in more than twenty international matches. Perhaps the name itself was banned by the eternally sanctimonious BBC.

Which brings me neatly on to one of the most memorable moments in Irish folklore. In 1985 Ireland were going for an historic Grand Slam against France at the old Lansdowne Road stadium in Dublin but the match will be forever recalled for a totally different reason. In the Irish team was another genial second row forward, the truly legendary Willie Anderson who had earlier been imprisoned for three months whilst on a 1978 tour in Buenos Aires for idiotically (or in true Irish fashion) trying to smuggle a flag from a government building. During this grudge match the TV camera man very observantly spotted a banner in the crowd proudly reading 'Our Willie is bigger than your Condom'.

On the same subject I have always been amused that the quaintly named French letters used to be translated as *les capotes Anglaises (carefully note the feminine)*. I think this delightful nuance in translation says far more about *l'Entente Cordiale* and the peculiar regard the French have for the English than thousands of astute analyses. For the record the modern French name for a condom is a *préservatif*, which is equally fitting if you think about. Another intriguing if less logical translation for a blow-job is to *faire le pompier*. Pretty insulting to a fireman I would have thought, but what would an innocent Englishman know about such deviant matters. For those who really want to understand the French psyche, compulsory reading is *The French* by the brilliant Theodore Zeldin, ironically himself a British citizen.

Where was I? Oh yes, Arthur Dailey or AD for short, but in no way to be confused with the ascetic and boring Adam Dagleish of dubious detective fame. Monsieur Lacapère had passed on to me a pleasant colonial couple because he was too *paresseux* (lazy) to work at weekends. As I had nothing suitable, in turn I passed them on to AD. The latter soon found them a nicely modernised stone property in the tiny commune of Bives and quickly nailed down a deal. By the saints he was like a benign tiger when a sale was in the offing. Of course the deal was '*en noire*' or under the table. Again people who haven't lived in France just can't comprehend in the slightest the French's singular aversion to paying taxes. To them it was just a *jeu*. I suppose the nearest equivalent we have in England would be tax avoidance (or rather evasion) schemes concocted by 'honourable' accountants. To my simple eyes I can't see much difference. It is a game played by everyone including *notaires*, who just turn a blind eye when assured there is no commission involved, or even as in one case I was involved in, actually leave the room so that cash can change hands. No names, no packdrill. Anyway as relations had rapidly deteriorated with M Van Gogh after he had realized that I wasn't an English goldmine I was buggered if I was going to pass on eighty per cent of my commission to him. And of course if I was to be honest, which I wasn't, I desperately needed every franc I could get my grubby hands on just to keep the creditors at bay and to stop the family from starving. To mélange Francis of Assisi and Somerset Maugham, Christ give me principles but not quite yet. It is only when your back is truly against the wall that your precious integrity is revealed as nothing more than a middle class malaise. Anyway the long and the short of it was that AD handed over twenty thousand *balles* (slang for francs) to me for about five minutes work after I had slogged over fourteen months for sod all. What an irony.

Seriously if anyone thinks estate agents commission is excessive I for one would be happy to work on a quantum meruit basis. Being the worst *agent immobilier* in France I would say that, wouldn't I? Of course the vendors would never wear it. Therefore the next time the GDP (Great British Public silly) bellyache, remember that realtors only get paid on results, unlike our legal brethren who get paid whether they get a result or not, and with money up front of course. If the English think they pay over the odds in commission they are in clover there compared to what goes on in France. The commission in the Gers was a pretty generous five to seven per cent whilst in the Vienne department near Poitiers, where I was later to be involved in a controversial sale, it rose to a usurious ten per cent. No wonder the French are even less keen to pay commission than the English and why there is so much litigation. On that latter subject I was very soon to have another 'interesting' case.

My riches didn't last very long, exacerbated by a very expensive wild goose chase (une chasse sauvage) all the way down to Biarritz about two hundred kilometers away looking for a piece of prime real estate for some cranky Yankee client. I was always looking for something on the distant horizon. I also seemed to attract more than my fair share of *promeneurs* (timewasters) who were either just on a reconnaissance trip or waiting to sell their house in England.

Coming to the end of the year I still had not brought any revenue to the greedy coffers of M Van Gogh and our relationship was already at breaking point before *l'affaire Masseng* broke in November. At last I had a promising Dutch photographic client who was very interested in a little wreck near Lectoure in the tiny village of Larroque Engalin. However negotiations were very tough and well matched between another cunning Gascon *paysan* and a typically flinty Dutchman. In the end with negotiations deadlocked I halved my own commission to seal the deal. To compensate for this I tried the trusty AD approach of getting the purchaser to pay me *en noire*. Of course I was as crappy at corruption as I was at selling and word leaked back to M Van Gogh via a nasty Lectoure *notaire* and he promptly threatened me with legal action. Having been well and truly caught with my probity pants down I had no choice but to capitulate ignominiously to him. However glorious revenge was exacted two years later when M van Gogh was caught by AD with his own pants literally down on the bed of the master bedroom of a property we were both trying to sell, with a new attractive female negotiator in tow as it were. Not much room for manoeuvre there.

Back to *l'affaire Masseng* which certainly wasn't a subject for any humour. As I had already halved my commission to close the deal I had brilliantly managed to obtain the worst of every world. Not only did I only get three thousand francs commission for all my hard work I had to concede seven thousand francs to the fat man. Even more galling, the latter received the total commission direct from the *notaire* whilst I had to grovel to M Van Gogh to even receive my measly share. Having got his pound of flesh he then had both might and right on his side in terminating my contract with him forthwith. The vicious sting in the tail was that he would now actively enforce the craftily inserted clause in my contract that specified I couldn't work again for a year within fifty kilometers of Fleurance. I was assured by the best legal brains available that the clause was strictly enforceable which meant that I wouldn't be able to work as an agent for the whole of 1993. I was fucked.

By this time we had officially closed the Auberge and the house had already been covertly on the market for over three months. Its rapid sale was now my only hope. In the meantime we sold the last of our valuable furniture and looked forward to a very Happy Christmas. Like hell we did but hell had to wait a little longer. My only memory of that disastrous non-festive holiday was a repeat on the TV of The Band's last concert in the memorable Martin Scorsese film The Last Waltz. The film included a callow Van Morrison doing an inspired version of his famous song Caravan.

'Turn up your radio and let me hear the song
Switch on your electric light
Then we can find out what is really wrong'.

But of course I couldn't and didn't. Neither had I involved or explained anything to my wife during this period. In fact she accused me on a number of occasions of not sharing my feelings with her but my only answer was always that I didn't have any feelings. This patently wasn't true. Of course I had bloody feelings. They seethed inside me till I was ready to explode. It was just that I wasn't ready to share them with anyone in the whole wide world, let alone my wife. I didn't want anyone to see inside my pathetic failure of a life. This naturally caused Mandy extreme frustration that I apparently regarded her from some detached position deep within me and she just couldn't penetrate these defences, even though these defences were more of a Maginot Line than a Rock of Gibraltar.

Chapter 4 – Golf and Gourmandise in Gascony

The first few months of 1993 passed in a daze. Doctor Bouchard from Saint Clar did his best but as I still couldn't or wouldn't tell him what was really wrong there was little he could do. He gave me some different drugs including Diazepam but they just made me feel even more of a zombie. Eventually in June we managed to sell Saint Martin via some fancy agents in Auch. How we lasted out that long with no income I just don't know. I do remember cashing in my Commercial Union life assurance policy that Dad had started for me in 1969 when I was twenty one and would reach maturity when and if I reached the right old age of sixty five in far off 2013. He had also paid the premium of £52 per annum ever since. The accumulative value in 1993 had already reached the amazing figure of over £8000 but when I cashed the policy in prematurely I only received about £2000. As I write this in the winter of 2010, that far off date of 2013 is now only round the corner and the nest egg that my father had far-sightedly set up for me would have amounted to a very tidy sum on full maturity. Ah yes, regrets I have had a lot and far too many to mention. At least I can console myself that I only sold my own family silver, so to speak, unlike that sagacious Mr Brown who flogged off all the nation's gold for a fistful of dollars.

The purchasers of Saint Martin were a pair of Parisian teachers who wanted it first as a holiday house and then to retire to in due course. The agents sensed my parlous position and ruthlessly beat me down from my very reasonable asking price of one million francs. Yes, Saint Martin would have been a brilliant investment for the future as well if I hadn't have been so broke and desperate. A decade later I broke a rule of a lifetime never to go back to a former home when we revisited the Gers on holiday. We stopped for a quick peek and were delighted to find that Saint Martin still had the same owners and that they hadn't been out to make a fast buck. The whole exterior of the property had been redecorated completely and it now gleamed pristine in the bright September sun. Not only that but they had also ripped out the massive terrace which had structurally destabilized the back of the house and put in a spanking new swimming pool to boot. It was now truly one of the finest houses in the area and I was proud to have made a little contribution along the way.

At the signing Max the *notaire* suggested that a friend of his in the *immobilier* trade might be interested in an association. Of course I didn't mention my ban and stirred myself enough to potter down to picturesque Sarrant near Beaumont to the rather menacing sounding *Donjon Immobilier*. Monsieur Rivière was a big, bluff straight talking *mec* (bloke) but he also seemed rather too sure of himself and it seemed I would be cast as a lowly negotiator again for the foreseeable future when my whole aim was to run my own agency eventually. I was so suspicious and apprehensive after my unfortunate experience with M Van Gogh that I adopted my normal Fabius Cunctator tactics when in doubt; that is delay, delay and then delay a bit more. I eased my conscience by saying to myself that I was banned from the *immobilier* trade anyway and there was nothing I could do about it. Of course I could have sought further legal advice on the ban but that would have required some effort. I therefore did nothing but laze in the sun like a now truly geriatric Graduate.

On the sale of Saint Martin we immediately bought another house, a much more modest affair reflecting our diminished circumstances, but not before a lot of resistance on my part. Mandy had originally sighted the property in question a year or so earlier amongst my agents photographs and immediately fallen in love with it. A true *coup de foudre* or love at first sight (literal translation flash of lightning). The house had the total opposite effect on me and I apparently described it 'as a shack' in a most derogatory manner. Of course it was still on the market and of course it was another cunning Gascon farmer we had to deal with. In the end AD managed to force a sale although the seller still had much the better of the deal, especially considering the house had been empty for some years and was in a dreadful state inside. In fact I wouldn't move in until Mandy and Daughter No 2 had carried out a massive preliminary clean up. The property was a low-slung stone house with *pigonnier* plus a large range of outbuildings and an acre of land. The hamlet was called Heuré-Bartens and the house bore the same name. It was situated near the village of Isle Bouzon between Saint Clar and Lectoure. Heuré could have made a superb property but needed a hell of a lot of money, work and vision to bring it up to scratch. Unfortunately I only had a little bit of money, little appetite for work and no vision. Mandy continued to work like a black Gascon in her spare time to get it into shape in as she had just started a job teaching English at one of the local schools during the day. Meanwhile I raised just enough energy to take up golf again. There was over a hundred thousand francs left over after the purchase of Heuré and I immediately blew five thousand francs of my new found wealth on a set of Ping Zing clubs. Oh yes, I was back in big spender mode again. I didn't get where I am today by saving or scrimping. I had hardly played golf for twenty years but spent the rest of the summer trying to make up for that legendary Moving Finger from Omar Khayyam. I joined the Lasalle club near Fleurance, where the *propriétaire* Gérard soon made me feel at home. It was only a tiny nine hole course but full of ups and downs with greens that would put many a major English club to shame. There were barely a hundred members with a hard core of about a dozen semi-professional players including myself.

First and foremost amongst these semi-professionals was the bombastic but charismatic Pierre Lagaillarde whose booming voice and staccato laugh could be heard two fairways away. He was supposedly a barrister at Auch, and apparently a former paratrooper and deputy to the National Assembly for Algiers in the distant past, who somehow contrived to play virtually every afternoon. He also mentioned casually to me during the course of a round one afternoon that there had once been a price on his head back in Algeria. What Pierre didn't mention was that his past was far more colourful and complicated than he let on. Pierre became a close friend and quietly assisted me in one or two of my dodgy legal altercations. He was apparently known as a *casse-tout*, or hellraiser, in his younger days in Algeria. On reading this line Mandy unhelpfully added that she could see now why we got on so well. Much, much more on the subject of Pierre Lagaillarde and *la guerre d'Algérie* in the next chapter.

For the record one million *pieds noirs* fled to France after the referendum to decide the future of the country and Algeria finally gained independence in July 1962 after eight years of a bloody civil war which made the Troubles in Northern Ireland look like a garden tea party. Almost a million native Algerians died in the conflict and around nine hundred French soldiers. The scars live on to this day. Perhaps our government got it right by negotiating with Mr Adams and the IRA after all, although I still find it difficult to reconcile the blanket amnesty for over a hundred murdering Irish terrorists. And if we are going to negotiate with terrorists in Northern Ireland, by the same principle why can't we negotiate with al-Qaeda? Answers on a post card to the coalition government, if they are still talking to each other.

Another semi-professional was Philippe despite ostensibly having something to do with pharmaceuticals. We also had the sinister Gilles *le Corse*, rumoured to be a debt collector. I wouldn't have fancied being pursued by him for any of my debts. Pierre and Gilles couldn't stand each other and Pierre paid him the ultimate insult in French by addressing him as *vous* instead of tutoying him as is normal when you know someone well. Except of course Giscard D'Estaing, the former French president, who was so old-fashioned that he even addressed his wife as *vous*. French is such a subtle language in so many respects. I knew I had been fully accepted at the golf club when I was asked to *tutoyer* them by my fellow golfers and also allowed to kiss all the lady players on meeting them. That was one of the many reasons I enjoyed playing golf so much in France. Green fees and membership was cheap and attire casual. You could wear jeans and tee shirts or whatever you liked, unlike in England with its stupid dress code. There you could dress like a prat in Pringle pullovers and ghastly trousers or boy scout shorts and that was OK, but wear expensive designer jeans and you were driven out of the club like a criminal. Women could also play with the men if you see what I mean, even though they were engaged in different competitions. I bought Daughter No 3 a mini set of clubs and she got very keen, but when she returned to England she was eventually put off completely after only being allowed to play with all the old ladies.

Another regular was *petit* Gilbert with a swing like a demented scythe, whilst his son Julian had a very elegant swing and played off a handicap of four. Young Patrice was the club's star player off two and another not so regular was Jean-Luc Arnaud, who was both the chef and owner of the magnificent *Hôtel de Bastard* at Lectoure which also offered the best cuisine in the Gers.

No mention of cuisine in the Gers would be complete without a little digression on that peculiarly French delicacy, foie gras. The Americans are always wittering on about the inhumanity of force feeding and their Food Police have even started to ban it in restaurants in some areas. As mentioned earlier no bird would submit unwillingly to *le gavage* if it was not a happy one so I would totally refute the wild accusations of cruelty. To give foie gras a further boost, recent studies have suggested it may offer those who eat it protection from heart disease. Whilst the rest of the overfed western world dutifully munches lean meats and unsaturated oils, the French, contrary as ever, continue to kick off a meal with the exorbitant and revered goose liver, dripping in calories and animal fat. It has all become known as *le paradox français*. For, despite this staunch display of dietary rebellion, the rate of heart disease in France happens to be the lowest in Europe and second only to Japan in the world.

How the French can eat a diet that is high in animal fat yet still manage to avoid heart disease is a mystery to scientists. Only 145 in every 100,000 middle-aged Frenchmen die of heart attacks annually. In pious America and Flora Britain, the toll is more than twice as high. But what baffles doctors even further is the fact that the area of France with the highest consumption of animal fat has an even lower rate than the national average. Dr Serge Rénaud, director of research at the *Institut National de la Santé et de la Récherche Medicale* in Lyon; recently reported the results of a 10-year study that looked at the eating habits and mortality rates of the south western province of Gascogne. The Gascons, producers of 80 per cent of the world's *foie gras*, eat a diet higher in animal fat than any other group of people in the industrialized world, claimed Dr Rénaud. Yet studies carried out by the World Health Organisation's Multinational Monitoring of Trends and Determinants in Cardiovascular Disease (yes really!) found that the Gascons also have the lowest rate of death from heart attacks and the longest life expectancy in the whole of France.

'We have always known that our diet is healthy', says Mr Justamus, the director of the local chamber of commerce, who eats around two kilos of foie gras a year. 'In Gascogne we know how to eat well, at times we have a little excess....but we maintain the *équilibre*.' He admits, however, that the relaxed lifestyle of Gascogne could also have something to do with the health and the longevity of its inhabitants. 'We have a tranquil life, without stress. We take time to live and to eat, as one should'.

American researchers have also suggested that the Gascogne recipe for tranquil living and good eating habits may be the solution to *le paradox français*. Could it be that *pâté de foie gras*, wine and a siesta are about to surpass skimmed milk, oatbran and exercise on the healthy heart recommendations? *Bon appétit.*

In the United States where avoiding animal fat has become as a holy war (and you know where that got us) as a dietary recommendation, such statistics are hard to swallow. What the Americans don't realize is that the structure of duck and goose fats are much closer in chemical composition to olive oil and contains more of the good monounsaturated and polyunsaturated fats which can reduce cholesterol. This says Dr Rénaud, makes it a much healthier choice than pork and beef pâtés, which are high in harmful saturated fats. Also bear in mind that the finest roast potatoes are those made with goose fat. *Bon appétit.*

Back to golf I soon got back to my former handicap of fourteen but could progress no further because of a suspect swing and an even more suspect temperament. When the going got tough I hit the rough, but luckily not in the same way as a fractionally more famous golfer did last year. I also got irritated by my playing partners lack of comprehension of my idiosyncratic version of Suffolk French until the day that Dennis the *agriculteur* told me about his son studying at some strange place in *Écosse* called Abba Din. It took four recounts before I realized that he was talking about Aberdeen. On the same subject of language problems I was playing one day with my usual four ball when we reached a tense moment on the seventh green. I muttered *je dois encuillir ce put* (I must hole this putt) and was somewhat mystified and miffed when the others all burst out in hysterics. It was only when I reported the incident to my precocious daughters that evening they pointed out the error of my ways. *Encuillir* had apparently come out as *enculer*, a Three Star Merde word not to be translated for a family publication. Luckily this is not a family publication so I can blushingly tell readers that I had said I must bugger this putt. To get my own back the next day I asked those smug bastards to try Portsmouth, Southampton and Worthing, followed up with Wiveliscombe for good measure. Fifteen forty perhaps?

There were three other main courses in the Gers. Isle Jourdain to the south west towards Toulouse was another tricky little nine hole course with a lot of water, whilst Auch was a tricked up eighteen hole hilly course with a number of silly and artificial holes. Eauze to the west of Condom was my favourite. It was a genuine eighteen hole course over lovely rolling countryside with lots of fabulous views.

Outside the Gers my favourite course was Seilh just to the north of Toulouse which was both long and wide open which suited my wayward game. I had two particularly interesting experiences there. The first one was when my partner for the day took an enormously powerful swing at the ball on the first hole and we all gazed into the distance to observe the ball, but it had disappeared completely. Eventually we looked down to the tee where the tip of the ball was just visible. He had only gone and smashed the ball underground. I have never seen that done before or since. The other experience was when I thought my luck was really in when I was paired with a particularly attractive blonde *mademoiselle*. Not so attractive was the torrent of filth that emanated from her pert mouth all afternoon. Pretty lips should be used to better effect. Unfortunately those little people in glass houses shouldn't throw stones and the truth of this proverb was brought home to me when Daughter No 2 refused to caddy for me any more because of my unpleasant behaviour on the course. Surely not trying to set an example to a certain Mr Woods but golf certainly brings out the worst in people. In my case things reached their nadir at Auch after I had done particularly well to reach one of the par fives in two. I had been playing badly up to that point and was in a foul mood so when one of my lady partners asked me if I was surprised to find the ball on the green, I snarled no, I expected to find it in the fucking hole. No trouble with my French there or its comprehension. Conversation was a bit subdued after that.

Another fine course was at Albi where I was playing with Gilles and Phillipe one golden January morning and hit one of the finest shots of my career. At the long par five dog leg fifth I deliberately hooked a drive round the dogleg to open up the green. From there I hit a magnificent five wood over water all the way right to the back of the green. From there my putt for an eagle lipped out and then my tiny return effort for a birdie missed as well. That was the story of my golfing life because I was in truth a truly crappy putter. That was the main difference of my play compared with Pierre because he was a wonderful putter with a unique reverse croquet stance. He also hit the ball remarkably straight and as befitting a former paratrooper, didn't seem to suffer any nerves about such trivial matters as getting a little white ball into a silly little hole. But there again, I never could keep things in proportion. The story of my life.

Chapter 5 : Pierre Lagaillarde et la Guerre d'Algérie

'In terms of the broad canvas of French affairs, the mad May days of 1958 seem to belong to a long past era: to the storming of the Bastille, to the revolutionary scenes of 1830 and 1848, to the tragic-comic extravaganzas of the Commune of 1871, rather than to contemporary history less than two decades old. The events in Portugal since April 1974 help make the sacking of the Gouvernement-Général office in Algiers, the invasion of Corsica, the threat of paras floating down on the French homeland itself, and the overthrow of the Fourth Republic all appear not quite so improbable as they might have done a few years previously. Yet still that final fortnight of May 1958 remains one of the most extraordinary and melodramatic interludes, intoxicated and intoxicating, that the modern European mind can recall, a work of the *romancie*r rather than that of the historian. Out of millions of words written about it, an immense confusion of acts, motives and men emerges.'

So wrote Sir Alistair Horne in his magisterial book 'A Savage War of Peace, Algeria 1954-1962'. The first men to emerge into this mayhem were 'The Group of Seven', who represented the most extreme *pied noir* factions. First and foremost of the Seven was Pierre Lagaillarde who would perform a key role in May 1958 and again during 'Barricades Week' in January 1960.

Born in France in 1931 in Corbevoie on the outskirts of Paris, Lagaillarde had passed most of his childhood in Blida, the second city of Algeria, where both his parents had practised law. But the forbear with whom Lagaillarde like most to identify himself was his great-grandfather who had found immortality in the 1851 uprising against Louis-Napoleon. Leaping on top of a barricade and shouting 'I'll show you how one dies for twenty-five sous a day', he had been promptly shot. Lagaillarde himself had returned to study law at Algiers University the previous autumn, having completed his military service as a *sous-lieutenant* with the paras. This had taken him to the Suez Canal disaster and through the bloody Battle of Algiers, and his commandant had been sufficiently impressed to invite him to stay on but he had been refused with the contemptuous rebuff: 'The paras have every physical courage, but no civil courage!' Nevertheless, he seldom missed an occasion to appear (improperly) in uniform. The Brombergers in their journalistic classic *Les 13 Complots du 13 Mai* described Lagailllarde as 'a character in search of an author, wanting to be a Siegfried or a D'Artagnan'. But with his tall, lean figure, carpet-fringe beard and unsmiling face, he ressembled more closely the 'Knight of the Sorrowful Countenance'. Frequently his gestures were neither less grandiloquent nor less absurd than Don Quixote's. But he was undoubtedly a man of action. At the university the staccato laugh and raucous, rabble-rousing oratory, as well as his sheer panache, had at once made him a natural leader.

Lagaillarde regarded the Gaullists with detached contempt, remarking at an early stage that he wanted 'to have nothing to do with the Punch-and-Judy coup d'état of M. Chauban-Delmas'. His fellow members of 'The Group of Seven' went even further in their antipathy to de Gaulle. In this they were representative of the deep-seated Pétainist inclinations of the *pied noirs*, inherited from the internal conflicts of French North Africa during the Second World War. The 'Seven' wanted the army to take over in Algeria to preserve L'*Algérie française*.

In the midst of all these shenanigans, the news on May 9th that three French soldiers had been executed by the insurgents shook Algiers to the very core. This led to a telegram from General Raoul Salan (the French

Commander-in-Chief in Algeria) to the Chief of the General Staff in Paris.

'The present crisis shows that the political parties are profoundly divided over the Algerian question. The Press permits one to think that the abandonment of Algeria would be envisaged in the diplomatic processes which would begin with negotiations aiming at a ceasefire.....

The army in Algeria is troubled by recognition of its responsibility towards the men who are fighting and risking a useless sacrifice if the representatives of the nation are not determined to maintain L'Algérie française....' (ring any bells?)

'I request you to bring to the attention of the President of the Republic our anguish, which only a government firmly determined to maintain our flag in Algeria can efface'.

It was a clear cut ultimatum. Virtually for the first time since Napoleon's coup of the 18th *Brumaire* a French army was about to interfere directly in national politics. Into this feverish atmosphere Lagaillarde now stepped forward.

'Tomorrow (May 13th), I am going to seize the radio and the Gouvernement-Général, and I shall throw the files out of the windows. We shall perhaps be shot up, but Salan will be obliged to take power. As for me, I swear that I shall not leave the demonstration before getting into Lacoste's office!'

Shortly after noon the next day Lagaillarde appeared at the *Otomatic* and dramatically announced to the students there: 'From now on I consider myself an insurgent'. At about four o'clock the now dense crowds thronging the approaches to the *monument* parted like the waters of the Red Sea as a grim-faced Lagaillarde, clad in full para regalia, strode through. Arriving at the *monument*, he leaped nimbly up on to the plinth and, flanked by other leaders of the 'Seven', vehemently harangued the crowd: 'Are you going to let L'*Algérie française* be sold down the river? Will you allow traitors to govern us? Will you go to the end of the line to keep L'*Algérie française?*' The massed *pied noirs* roared back their approval. The mob surged up to the forum and then on into the Governor-General's grandiose office. In a matter of moments Lagaillarde was realising his ambition of the night before. Students appeared at every window, flinging out sheaves of documents and dossiers. Standing on the roof of the central balcony that was to become the focus of world attention over the next few days, Lagaillarde was greeted in the midst of this snowstorm by the wildest applause.

The invasion by the mob, the volleys of paper streaming from the 'G-G' windows, all bore an extraordinary resemblance to that other bizarre episode in French history – the seizure of the *Hôtel de Ville* by the Paris Communards in 1870. So did the scenes that followed. A young man in glasses pushed himself forward and when asked for his name, replied 'André Baudier, clerk in council housing....'

'But who do you represent?'

'The mob!'

Colonel Jaques Massu (commander of the élite 10th Para division) dutifully wrote down Baudier at the top of his list. Then came Lagaillarde, followed by a series of *illustres inconnus* drawn from the crowd. Announcing the formation of the Committee of Public Safety, Massu received a rapturous reception from the crowd outside. Almost as an afterthought, three Muslin worthies representing nine million Algerians were added to the list.

Later that night the Gaullists adroitly turning the situation to their advantage and prevailed upon Salan to send a new and crucial message to President Coty stating, 'the responsible military authorities esteem it an imperative necessity to appeal to a national arbiter with a view to constituting a new government of national safety. A call for calm by this high authority is alone capable of re-establishing the situation'. Salan, cautious as ever, had expunged from the original draft the name of de Gaulle, but the reference to 'a national arbiter' and 'this high authority' was explicit enough. At the same time a direct appeal was sent to de Gaulle himself. The cat was out of the bag, the army of Algeria had at last committed itself.

The 14th was a black day for the leaders inside the 'G-G' as de Gaulle had still not come forward. In Algiers the next day Salan appeared once more on the 'G-G' balcony before the ever present crowds in the Forum below. He spoke in moving tones of his attachment to the soil of Algeria and added: 'What has been done here will show to the world that Algeria wants to remain French. Our sincerity will carry with us all Moslems'. He concluded his address with a vibrant 'Vive la France! Vive l'Algérie française! Et vive de Gaulle!'

Sparked by Salan's utterance, de Gaulle now came out of his hermit crab shell for the first time. Using carefully measured words, he declared to the nation that 'in the face of the trials that are again mounting towards it, it should know that I am now ready to assume the powers of the republic'. But there was no how or when. As Prime Minister Macmillan noted sardonically in his journal, it was 'an equivocal statement, but one which has terrified the French politicians. It is cast in his usual scornful but enigmatic language'.

In Algiers, however, de Gaulle's declaration was greeted with the wildest enthusiasm. The following day, May 16th, the euphoria of the moment occasioned one of the most remarkable occurrences of the whole war. *Pieds noirs* linked arms with the Moslems, European girls lifted the veils of acquiescent Muslim women and all together sang the *Marseillaise* and the military *Chant des Africains*. Heady new slogans of 'From Dunkirk to Tamanrasset, fifty five million French', passed amongst the crowd. Suddenly the horrors of the Milk-Bar and Casino bombings, of the backlash *ratonnades* (Arab killings), seemed all but forgotten.

Historians still find the 'fraternisation' phenomenon of May 16th hard to explain. Stern critics of *L'Algérie française* like *Le Monde* and Francois Mauriac agreed on the genuineness of the demonstration, acclaiming it as a basis for new optimism. However disillusion was bound to follow on both sides as euphoria was replaced by the realisation that the fraternisers were still worshipping different gods. Nevertheless, as in that other dawn celebrated by Wordsworth, it was bliss to be alive in Algiers on that day of May 16th, and for a brief spell it looked as if all might be possible; so long as de Gaulle would grasp the nettle.

In Paris tension was mounting and seventy American tourists refused to leave their plane at Orly for fear of being caught up in a revolution. Then, on the afternoon of the 19th, de Gaulle summoned a press conference at the Palais d'Orsay.

Events in Algeria, he declared had indeed led to 'an extremely grave national crisis.... but this could also prove to be the beginning of a kind of resurrection.' Almost with modesty he added that was why 'the moment seemed to me to have come when it would be possible for me once again to be directly useful to France'. Though he praised the army in Algeria, he pointedly omitted any reference to an Algerian solution as such; an omission which was only to attain full significance in later years. All that was made crystal clear was that his price for returning was, as it always had been, the abolition of the political system of the Fourth Republic as it stood. Everything else had to be inferred. He ended: 'Now I shall return home to my village and there hold myself at the disposition of the country'.

The precise formula for his return was to be left to lesser mortals.

In Algiers de Gaulle's press conference was greeted with a mixture of satisfaction and impatience. Time was clearly against the 'revolt' in its increasing isolation, and the unhurried stance of de Gaulle was more than vexing. Therefore plans were initiated for a military intervention in France to force the hand of both the government and the slow moving de Gaulle. Conceived by Massu, it was eventually code-named 'Résurrection' which was stolen from the phrase used by de Gaulle at his press conference. The date provisionally fixed for *'Résurrection'* was the 27th-28th, with Massu declaring confidently in a press interview on May 23rd that: 'In eight days, General de Gaulle will be in power'.

On May 24th an astonished France learned that Massu's paras had seized power in Corsica. The coup was carried out by the 11th Shock without a shot being fired. When asked by journalists if there had been any casualties, Pascal Arrighi, the Gaullist deputy for Corsica who had taken part in the operation, contemptuously replied: 'Of course not! It was a revolution, not an election!'

On the morning of the 27th the crisis reached its peak. Parisians looked up nervously at every plane passing overhead and in the Ministry of the Interior Jules Foch received an intelligence report that *'Résurrection'* was now scheduled to take place on the following night. He ordered his C.R.S. force to prepare to defend government buildings. Meanwhile young para officers were arriving in the capital in civilian clothes carrying suspiciously heavy suitcases. Among their targets was the kidnapping of Jules Foch himself, and with them, on his own mission, came Lagaillarde. Then, early in the afternoon, de Gaulle, apparently as a result of the mounting pressures on him, issued a communiqué announcing that he had begun the 'regular process' of forming a new government. At the same time he sent a signal to Salan in which he called for the dropping of all thoughts of *'Résurrection'*. In Algiers Salan was manifestly delighted to be let off the hook, and despatched his deputy on a liaison mission to Columbey-les-deux-Églises. There de Gaulle spelled out to him in the clearest terms yet:-

'I want to be summoned as an arbiter coming at the demand of the whole country, to take over direction of a country so as to spare it useless rendings. I must appear as the man of reconciliation and not as the champion of one of the factions confronting each other'.

In Paris there was widespread jubilation and relief. Maurice Schumann was heard to exult: 'He's won. We've won. France has won.'

On the night of the 28th a fresh constitutional impasse threatened and de Gaulle told the Assembly that if they backed Le Troquer, the Leader of the Assembly, then 'I shall have no alternative but to let you have it out with the paratroops, while I go back into retirement and shut myself up with my grief.' Meanwhile a fresh ultimatum had reached President Coty from Algiers; either it was de Gaulle by 15.00 hours on the 29th, or *'Résurrection'* would go in at 01.00 hours the following morning. After a sleepless night, President Coty took a decision of tremendous guts when he announced the next morning that he had himself invited de Gaulle to form a government and that if this were rejected by the Assembly he would resign. The President's announcement 'tolled the knell', said de Gaulle, and on the 30th he agreed to form a government and a long sigh of relief swept over France.

On Sunday June 1st de Gaulle presented himself to the National Assembly, the first time he had entered it since January 1946 and was voted into power by 329 to 224 votes. De Gaulle was manifestly unhappy at being unable to obtain a bigger majority. Also disappointed were

Lagaillarde and the several hundred 'volunteers' from Algiers hovering in the bistros near the government quarter and awaiting orders to move in. They would be even more disappointed when the list of de Gaulle's first cabinet members was released. The Gaullist era had begun.

We next pick up the story of Pierre Lagaillarde and *la guerre d'Algérie* almost two years later. Entering its sixth year, the war had already lasted longer than the First World War and, as the new year of 1960 approached, it was about to bring with it events that would seal the fate of *Algérie française*.

Since well before de Gaulle's recent 'self determination' speech of September 16th, 1959, opposition to him had been steadily mounting among the ranks of *pied noir* 'ultras', increasingly distrustful of the policy of the man they considered they had brought back in May 1958. Lagaillarde, the would be d'Artagnan, had been elected to the Assembly that November, and had partially withdrawn from the Algerian scene. In his absence Jo Ortiz, the flamboyant owner of the Bar du Forum, had moved in. Ortiz had chosen the fourth anniversary of the war, November 1st 1958, to launch a new body, the Front National Français (F.N.F.), embracing under one militant organisation all the various 'ultra' groupings. Behind Ortiz there now emerged another new and even more influential figure, Jean-Jaques Susini. There could hardly have been more contrasting figures than the two F.N.F. leaders. Ortiz, the burly, bonhomous bar-keeper with his hooked, prize-fighter nose, whose swarthy features and well-cut suits testified to his Spanish origins, epitomised the *pied noir* with his emotional vehemence. On the other hand, Susini, ugly and emaciated, was a cold fish but a fine speaker with brilliant political acumen. The two were admirably complementary to each other.

One of the more surprising aspects of this period was the way in which the army command permitted the creation of such a Frankenstein monster as the F.N.F. under its very nose. Ultimately blame must attach to General Maurice Challe, the new Commandant-in-Chief, for allowing such a concentration of armed power to build up under the sway of such a loose canon as Ortiz.

Massu had recently been promoted to be the super prefect of Algiers city. He claimed that he was 'the lid on the Algiers cauldron' and was confident that he could contain the pressure exerted by the simmering 'ultras'. He even felt that Lagaillarde was sufficiently in his pocket for him to invite the young deputy to join him at a Beethoven concert on January 13th, although Paul Delouvrier, the new Delegate–General (a less imposing title than Governor-General), had warned him in prophetic terms: 'General, you think you control these people but watch out. The day will come when they will declare to you: We are at the mercy of our troops; we have to march, will you march with us?'

Because of the intriguing of two of his colonels on whom he most depended, Massu was in fact being hoodwinked. Worse was to come when he plunged headlong into a tiger trap laid by a West German correspondent, Hans Ulrich Kempski, where he was suckered into stating on the record that 'We no longer understand the policy of General de Gaulle. Our greatest disappointment has been to see him become a man of the left. Myself, and the majority of the officers of command, will not execute unconditionally the orders of the Head of State.'

Far from being the 'lid', Massu provided that extra head of steam to blow up the whole cauldron. France was staggered; it was unbelievable that such damning criticism should have come from the faithful *grognard*, Massu, of all people. A furious de Gaulle announced that he had been 'insulted' by Massu and that he should be relieved of his post forthwith and summoned back to Paris. Even after all his top advisors and generals had pleaded one after another the danger that the sacking of Massu could create, de Gaulle refused to back down. When Challe prophesied that 'Blood will flow in Algiers,' he was told 'You exaggerate'. 'When thrown into a red hot boiler', said the Brombergers, 'a bucket of water does not appease the furnace. It unleashes an explosion of fire. The recall of Massu was the bucket of water thrown onto the Algiers furnace.'

Ortiz now had his green light. The moment the news came through on the evening of January 22nd that Massu was permanently banished, the F.N.F. announced that a general strike would begin on Sunday, the 24th. Because of his departure for the Chamber of Deputies and his ensuing split with Ortiz, Lagaillarde had been deliberately excluded from all preliminary councils of war. According to the latter at his subsequent trial, he knew nothing of what was afoot until rumours reached him at a café on the Saturday morning. This was not strictly true. Typically, he had already jumped the gun the previous evening by seizing a building within the university perimeter. With a handful of armed henchmen he had turned this into the first barricaded camp, bluntly informing the authorities that if anyone approached within thirty metres they would be fired upon, and that he would not quit the university until de Gaulle had yielded. Henceforth, right through the following week, there would not be one but two leaders and two camps, and to the very end Lagaillarde's would prove the more orderly.

A far darker shadow from Ortiz's point of view was the ambiguous stance of the army. Partly egged on by the earlier assurance given by the dissident colonels, partly deluded by his own méditerranéen-et-demi optimism, Ortiz had persuaded himself and his followers that once they had moved, the army would give virtually total support. Now, at the eleventh hour, Ortiz was told that the feeling of the army in general was that they would not fire on him, but on the other hand, they would not countenance a putsch.

For Ortiz however, it was too late to back off and on the morning of the 24th he set up a 'command post' at the *Compagnie Algérienne* in readiness.

Meanwhile Challe, at last appreciating the explosiveness of the situation, had taken his own precautionary measures. Realising that Lagaillarde could not now be dislodged from the university, nor Ortiz's men disarmed without bloodshed, he first threw roadblocks across all the routes into the city and then ordered all available gendarmes to be concentrated in and around the Gouvernement-Général to prevent any recurrence of Lagaillarde's coup of May 13th 1958. Reluctantly Colonel Debrosse, the commander of the gendarmes, was also forced to call for reinforcements from the 10th Para division for what he scathingly called 'a little local excitement'.

By mid afternoon the *Plateau des Glières* was packed with demonstrators estimated at thirty thousand strong. At Ortiz's 'command post' there was chaos reminiscent of the headier days of the Paris Commune. In the street below some young members of the F.N.F. began spontaneously to prise up paving stones and create a barricade.

Confronted by the challenge of the barricades now busily under construction Challe had to act. A concerted operation was ordered whereby the demonstrators were to be herded, gently but firmly, like driven game towards the west of the city whence most of them had come. Perhaps this was to be the first known sighting of 'kettling'? The plan depended upon a precisely co-ordinated movement in which the gendarmes under Debrosse would advance down the steps from the Forum towards the sea while at the same time the paras were to come in from the north and east.

At 18.00 hours the gendarmes began to move down the steep slope to the Forum. It was already getting dark when suddenly a couple of pistol shots rang out of the gloom. As if it were a signal, volleys of automatic fire from windows and rooftops opened up on the unfortunate gendarmes. Caught at a terrible disadvantage they fell like flies.

And where were the paras?

It was 18.45 before the advance guard of the paras arrived having taken the best part of an hour to cover six hundred yards. The shooting died slowly away but when the casualties came to be counted there were six dead and twenty four wounded among the civil demonstrators and no less than fourteen dead and one hundred and twenty three wounded in the ranks of the gendarmes. A violent exchange now took place between the para colonel and Debrosse, with the latter demanding why the paras had not turned up on time, and the colonel riposting that the gendarmes by opening fire had breached Challe's 'pact' with Ortiz. To this day, despite the lengthy hearings of the 'Barricades Trial' later in 1960, the essential question of who fired first has never been satisfactorily answered. Ring any bells? Hint Londonderry 1972.

Whatever the findings of any post mortem, a catastrophic frontier in the Algerian war had been crossed. For the first time Frenchmen had fired upon, and killed, other Frenchmen. Across the breadth of France there echoed the dying words of an Algerian gendarme: 'For two years I have been fighting against the *fellagha* (Arab guerrilla). Now I'm dying at the hands of the people who cry L'*Algérie française*! I don't understand....!'

Shattered by events and by the realisation of his own impotence, Challe made a stern broadcast declaring a state of siege over the city. But it had a minimal effect on either the insurgents or the sympathetic para colonels, all of whom were convinced that the day was won and that de Gaulle would have to give way.

On the Monday morning (January 25th) Ortiz was comporting himself like a triumphant pocket Duce. There was a brief fiery exchange with Lagaillarde, who habitually referred contemptuously to the restaurateur's disorderly 'command post' as *le café*, after which each retired to rule his own roost. Later that day Ortiz was heard to proclaim jubilantly: 'Tomorrow in Paris I will be the ruling power!'

But the jubilant Ortiz reckoned without the will of one man; de Gaulle.

When the first news reached France, ordinary Frenchmen did not take in at first just how dangerous the situation was in Algeria. However, from the very first de Gaulle displayed the same Olympian calm as during the explosive days of May 1958. In a short, unbending broadcast to the nation, he accused the Algerian insurgents of striking 'a stab in the back for France, before the world.' He adjured them to return to order. He went on to say that he had been brought back to lead the country, to find for Algeria *'une solution qui soit française'* and he intended to carry through this responsibility. As he wrote in his memoirs: 'I was determined to lance the abscess, make no concessions whatsoever and obtain complete obedience from the army.' He also refused to accede to pressure to bring forward the date of a television address he was to make to the nation, already fixed for Friday, January 29th. Even the loyal courtier, Bernard Tricot, admits that at the time he felt that de Gaulle's intransigence was due more to 'pride than careful calculation'. The whole entourage was in despair at what seemed like his withdrawal from reality. Yet, in fact, events were to prove that it was de Gaulle who was instinctively and accurately in touch with the mood of France. With the passing of each day of the crisis, it became evident that public opinion, from Left to Right, was getting solidly behind de Gaulle and solidly against the Algiers insurgents and the dissident colonels.

By the 27th, realization of this vital fact began to dawn upon these colonels in Algiers, with the more radical of them assessing that they had now missed the boat in not launching a full scale putsch during the first hours of the barricades. Bored with the discomfort behind Ortiz's barricades, some of his forces began to fritter away. Lagaillarde, always in his para's 'leopard' battle denims and red beret, continued to maintain strict military discipline in his camp. Confidently he declared to the press: 'The Third Republic was born at Sedan and died in Sedan. The Fourth was born in Algiers and died in Algiers. The Fifth is born in Algiers.' But there was no news that a single officer, let alone unit, of the army had come out in support of the insurgents. However, headed by Argoud, the most articulate of the 'Soviet of Colonels', they now made a last minute bid to persuade Challe and Delouvrier to join their cause and force de Gaulle to conform or go.

The thinly veiled threat that he and the Commander-in-Chief might soon find themselves little better than prisoners in their own headquarters helped decide Delouvrier to take a dramatic step; namely to leave Algiers, together with Challe. Perversely the news that the 'authorities' had withdrawn from Algiers produced an unexpectedly powerful effect on the insurgents, and was to mark a turning point in 'Barricades Week'. More of the *pied noir* militiamen began to disappear from Ortiz's barricades. Then on Friday the 29th the skies darkened in Algiers and rain began to patter down on the over-heated citizenry.

That night at eight o'clock, de Gaulle made his long-awaited television appearance. He first of all firmly repeated his September decision that 'the Algerians shall have free choice of their destiny'. Next he turned to the army, for whose benefit he had donned his own uniform that night, speaking in the most severely paternal terms:-

'What would the French army become but an anarchic and absurd conglomeration of military feudalisms, if it should happen that certain elements make their support conditional?   As you know, I have the supreme responsibility. It is I who bear the country's destiny. I must therefore be obeyed.   This having been said, listen to me carefully.....no soldier, under penalty of being guilty of a serious offence, may associate himself at any time, even passively with the insurrection.   In the last analysis, law and order must be re-established..... your duty is to bring this about. I have given, and am giving, this order.'

After a loaded pause, de Gaulle's harsh tone gave way to an imploring appeal: 'Finally, I speak to France. Well, my dear country, my old country, here we are together, once again, facing a harsh test. If I were to yield to the guilty ones, who dream of being usurpers, then France would become but a poor broken toy adrift on the sea of hazard'.

It was one of de Gaulle's finest speeches, a performance of hypnotic wizardry.   The impact on Frenchmen of all walks of life throughout France was nothing short of sorcery. As Bernard Tricot murmured to himself: *'C'est gagné.'*

It was indeed won, though the barricades dragged on for another forty eight hours.   Morale slumped as the rain continued to lash down. Inside the headquarters of Ortiz and Lagaillarde, an atmosphere resembling the Twilight of the Gods prevailed.   On January 30th,   A last bitter, reproachful encounter took place between the two leaders. Ortiz, utterly exhausted, accused the army of betrayal and Lagaillarde of being a maniac. The latter, contemptuous of Ortiz, 'that dish-wipe', declared that he himself would never surrender. In the end Delouvrier used Colonel Dufour, the officer most respected by Lagaillarde, to 'negotiate terms'. By the following night a most remarkable 'deal' had been concluded. Lagaillarde's men would be permitted to march out as 'soldiers', bearing arms, and would be accorded full honours by Dufour's paras. There would be a free pardon for all, except for the leaders of the insurrection. They were to surrender themselves to French justice.

By Monday morning, February 1st, Ortiz had vanished, never to be seen in Algiers again. But at midday Lagaillarde marched out with flags flying and in full military order. In a brief speech to his supporters he said: *'Ne regrettez rien.* You can't win them all, but a man is never vanquished when he retains deep within himself the will to fight.' He embraced his father and was then flown off to the Santé prison. Alain de Sérigny, who later joined him there on account of the support his *Écho d'Alger* had given the insurgents, declared perhaps extravagantly: 'If there was one man in this sinister affair, it was he, and if there was any grandeur, it was on his side.'

However, in spite of the above we are still not quite finished with *Pierre Lagaillarde et la Guerre d'Algérie.* At the long-awaited 'Barricades Trial', which started in November 1960 and lasted three months, sentences were surprisingly mild. Lagaillarde, bombastic as ever in front of the court, and demanding that his 'more distinguished actions' of May 1958 be taken into account, was given ten years, but placed at provisional liberty, from which he promptly absconded. Ortiz was sentenced to death in absentia while Susini, despite jumping bail, received no more than a two year suspended sentence.

In April 1961 Lagaillarde suddenly turned up in Madrid, together with Susini. The generals were plotting another putsch and restlessly searching for a leader while Salan (the 'Mandarin') had already set up court at the Hotel Princesca, also in Madrid. The 'Mandarin' was immediately alienated by the extravaganzas of Lagaillarde. 'I would indeed like to be shot,' the latter declared, 'but I want a general at my side!' His horizons were rising rapidly. He produced ideas for a full-scale reform of the army, gave a large cocktail party for the France-Spain football match, and expressed positive disappointment that he had been sentenced to only ten years (in absentia) at the 'Barricades Trial'. On hearing of this comment Salan's loyal adjutant, Captain Ferrandi, commented witheringly, that 'is really very little for a future head-of-state!' Salan was soon barely on speaking terms with Lagaillarde, and determined to exclude him at all costs from any military coup. Undeterred Lagaillarde and Susini sat down to devise a new body which, composed of civilians and military deserters, would continue to fight for L'*Algérie française* by underground techniques of terrorism. After some discussion they decided upon the title of *Organisation Armée Secrète*: O.A.S. When the details were reported to the 'Mandarin', he sighed contemptuously: 'Poor *pieds noirs*! They've already had the U.S.R.A.F., the F.A.F. and the F.N.F.! Now with this O.A.S. they will never be able to recognise it! Nevertheless, if it amuses them and helps them pass the time waiting for better things, then let them get on with it.'

When the putsch belatedly took place, Lagaillarde was prevented by the Spanish police from joining the party. The putsch had to do without its 'd'Artagnan'. And it didn't manage very well in the event, effectively defeated by another coruscating de Gaulle broadcast to the nation. One amusing off-shoot was the conduct (or rather lack of it) of the navy during the attempted coup. Admiral Querville had escaped to a warship and steamed off to the impregnable naval base of Mers-el-Kèbir. As one officer remarked acidly, 'It's always missed the boat, ever since Trafalgar!'

However, despite Salan's cynicism, the O.A.S. were to play a devastating and deadly role in events after the collapse of the putsch. In the event, Lagaillarde continued to remain in Spain but declared his readiness to return to Algeria and join the O.A.S. provided its senior leaders would 'write him personally an invitation in good and correct form'. Unfortunately they never did and Pierre

Lagaillarde was eventually arrested in Madrid and exiled to the Canary Isles only to be found over thirty years later on the rather more tranquil fairways of Gascony.

Chapter 6 – Dungeons, Germans and the Planet

Come December 1993 I was still in a state of mental flux even if I was in much better physical shape after all my golf. Then in a flash of inspiration I decided to have another go with Monsieur Rivière. *Donjon Immobilier* had by this time moved to the afore-mentioned Isle Jourdain with its watery golf course which was ideal for me because I could again mix business with pleasure. This time we quickly reached a very amicable agreement and I was to start work on January 1st, 1994, the day my ban with *SARL Immobilier* Van Gogh officially ended. Although my VW Golf was still going well I thought that a smart agent needed a smart car so I bought a brand new smart black Opel Corsa. Mini delusions of grandeur still persisted and I beat off Mandy's protests with my usual silky arguments that I knew she couldn't counter. Like I never took *Heuré* to my heart, so Mandy firmly refused to accept the Corsa as a permanent feature. She tells me to this day that she still looks at all black Corsas with distaste and a desire to distance herself, but of course I never listened at the time. In the event she had her wish, the Corsa didn't last very long. Perhaps it was jinxed or just damned.

Anyway, on I ploughed and put down fifteen thousand francs in cash with the remainder on HP at fifteen hundred francs a month. As I still had fifty thousand francs left over from the sale of Saint Martin, I thought that would give me an adequate cushion till I started earning again. Some hope as I hadn't made any money yet in France after almost five years and soon found out that Donjon had a poor range of properties and clients despite M Rivière's bullishness. I therefore had to build up my own portfolio of properties round Saint Clar and cultivate a few clients, which I did almost exclusively by bringing them in from the

UK with expensive advertising. I again had some promising nibbles, none more appetizing than an ambiguous lady of a certain age who put me immediately on my guard when she insisted on me inspecting her nice rented apartment near Auch. This would have been fine if it wasn't for the lacy black underwear draped suggestively in the bedroom. However like a true blue boy scout I was always well prepared and carefully inserted my box before our next appointment at a very remote location. In the event I retained my extra-marital virginity as she was this time far more stimulated by the historic *Château de Puyssentut*. Unfortunately the vendor, my golfing friend Dennis the *agriculteur*, got too greedy for his old wreck when it came down to the wire and it all fizzled out.

Another early client was the eccentric but amiable Peter Jamieson who specialized in testing my patience by always ringing first thing on a Saturday morning with no prior warning. He had sold his business on the Isle of Jersey and had apparently spent most of his recent past walking the world. He had a battered old Range Rover, a battered face and battered knees befitting an *ancient* (former not ancient) rugby player. He was also a fanatical ecologist and anguishedly bemoaned the ruthless use of weedkiller and lack of hedgerows throughout the Gers. Anyway we toured the *département* discussing rugby, pollution and generally putting the country to rights. We also enjoyed the odd beer or three together including a memorable session at Vic, or Vic Fezansac to the uninitiated, the Gersois capital of bullfighting. I think the gendarmes are still looking for him in connection with some confusion over an unpaid hotel bill at Fleurance. Interpol have not yet been informed as far as I know although he was once stopped and searched for drugs in the Pyrenees near the Spanish border on account of his suspicious looking vehicle and bohemian appearance, including long length army regulation war shorts issue. He used to appear out of the blue every six months or so. I don't think he ever had any intention of actually buying a property in

France but he was always an amusing and entertaining companion. He appeared for the last time after I had returned to England and Mandy said he seemed quite put out that I wasn't there to accompany him around as usual. By the way Peter, I would greatly appreciate it if you could return the book *'Planet under Stress: The Challenge of Global Change' (1990)* which you borrowed from me all those years ago. It was both edited and signed for me by my uncle, the late Dr Digby J. Mclaren, the distinguished Canadian geologist and palaeontologist. He later became better known as a crusader for political action to safeguard the planet's resources. In this respect he was years ahead of his time before climate change recently became fashionable for politicians, although Copenhagen has exposed both their lack of sincerity and the will to overcome the greatest challenge of our age. As he wrote in the preface to *Planet under Stress*:-

'The Royal Society of Canada began to focus its interest in Global Change in 1984. It also realized that perhaps the most important task was to inform the public as fully as possible on current research into global change, on the significance of the results as they are currently being interpreted, and on the social, economic, legal, and moral aspects involved in coming to terms with the most serious threat ever to have arisen to the healthy functioning of the planet, the home and support of humankind.

The human being is an animal that has moved out of ecological balance with its environment. Humankind is a wasteful killer and a despoiler of other life on the planet. The normal and apparently acceptable behaviour has been licensed by a belief that our use of the Earth's resources is God-given, and encourage by an economic system that place short-term profit as a benefit. We are only slowly learning to put a real cost on the resources we consume, and the wastes we produce. Humankind is now dominant in effecting perhaps irreversible change on the Earth's surface, and I suggest that we do not know enough to decide how we run this planet.'

He concluded the preface apocalyptically that 'All people on Earth are in this together, and so we must find a joint solution. It is too late to build walls around, or put roofs over, regions of the world. The problems are exclusively global, and the solutions must be also. We are now faced with a task that is more difficult than anything we have ever contemplated: to decide how we may continue to live on this small planet. Any departure from ecological balance that destroys most of the remaining life on earth - and the big killing is under way- will mean that we are doomed to a similar fate. In other words, it is imperative that we learn to live in balance with all of Earth's complexities. Humankind has never before been faced so urgently with such a challenge - but face it we must, or life on this planet, for human beings, may become insupportable.'

Digby's hopes of seeing fossil fuels phased out in his lifetime were not fulfilled, although he had way back in 1986 played a leading role in initiating the International Geosphere-Biosphere programme because of the threat of climatic warning. Such ideas were not 'crackpot' or the 'starry-eyed ramblings of do-gooders', he thundered: 'Unless we realise we are a piece of this planet we are doomed'. A veritable Nostradamus and a fine man, but my abiding memory of him was during a visit he made to Saint Martin with his wife Phyl when he 'blessed the carrots' in a noble attempt to entice Daughter No 3 to eat at least one type of vegetable. He is commemorated by the prestigious Digby Maclaren Medal of the International Commission in Stratigraphy and was able to attend the first inauguration in Florence shortly before his death in 2004.

Peter, the fine for the almost posthumous return of Digby's book has now amounted to the stiff penalty of three crates of Pelforth Brune with liquid interest still accruing and I look forward to hearing from you again at your very earliest convenience.

One of the main attractions of the new Corsa was its excellent radio. Test Match Special had recently switched to Radio 4 and the reception was remarkably good. I had been out of the cricket scene for five years now and was hungry to get back in touch, probably hungrier than I was to actually sell any houses. Therefore on another of my mad long distance visits across country into the Landes department in a misguided search for business, I had the greatest of pleasure of hearing South Africa making their long awaited return to Test cricket. Remarkably two of the promising young players who I had seen play for Western Province in Cape Town all those years ago in the mid seventies were now in the South Africa side, namely Kepler Wessels and Peter Kirsten. I fanatically followed the series through to the Oval where Malcolm Devon famously blitzed the Springboks.

That was the trouble. I was always being sidetracked into pleasant if unprofitable cul de sacs. By the way a cul de sac in French is a *voie sans issue*. Only the English could translate arse-sacking so ineptly. By June several promising clients and properties had disappeared into the *canicule* (heatwave). Somehow I kept my cool, and my swing, and was rewarded for my patience with Herr Hans. Earlier in the year I had placed a tiddly ad in the late but not lamented European newspaper. Of course this newspaper had previously been owned by Robert Maxwell, again late and again not lamented. More of him later. I was staggered to receive a phone call soon afterwards from a lady in Australia. I duly sent off a few details and didn't think any more about it. Then in late June I received another phone call from her saying her husband, Herr Hans, was on his way from Sydney via his native Germany. A week later I picked him up from Montauban station. He was short, bearded and with excess baggage both in his hands and round his waist. He was also sweating profusely. He didn't have a word of French and he didn't look like Goldfinger either. He was probably my most unlikely buyer ever which shows why I was such a lousy estate agent. His first needs were a beer, a TV and then a bed, strictly in that order. The World Cup had just started and he didn't want to miss another Teutonic victory. After several more beers I limped home somewhat worse for wear. It sure was a dirty job being an *agent immobilier* but someone had to do it. The two things you needed most were staying and drinking power. No problem with the latter. The next day we set off smoothly in AD's air conditioned Merc. At six o'clock we were tired and dishevelled having found nothing remotely satisfactory amongst numerous wrecks. Then AD had a final piece of inspiration and we whizzed off to the village of Le Sauvetat just west of Fleurance and *enfin trouvé une maison habitable*. Friday morning, only thirty six hours after Hans' arrival, the deal was signed and sealed. It also left me with another ten thousand *balles* in my back pocket. And twenty four hours later when Germany were knocked out of La Coupe Mondiale by Bulgaria, my cup truly ranneth over. I would explain in mitigation for this apparent disgraceful racial prejudice that I am not anti-German, just anti-German footballers ever since that heartbreaking defeat in Mexico in 1970. I am very much pro Angela Meikel and Bernhard Langer, especially when the latter is playing in the Ryder Cup, but from Herr Muller to Roomyknickers to Clansman, their footballers give me the coolies. If they had won the World Cup again that year I would have been forced to admit that first, there was a god after all, and second that he was German.

On to more serious matters. Just after Hans departure I was passed on a client from another English agent who worked in the south of the Gers near Mirande. The client was looking for a profitable arable farm but the only ones I had on my books were of little appeal. It was then that I applied those little grey cells again. If only I had applied them more often it could have all turned out so differently.

If, if if. Anyway I toddled down to the SAFER office at Auch to find something more appropriate for my client, Mr Mossman. The above acronym is short for *Société Aménagement Foncier et d'Etablissement Rural* and it is a quasi government organisation entitled to exert pre-emptive rights on the acquisition of farms or farmland. They are involved in all sales of land in France above two hectares and therefore wield a lot of fire power. They can block any sale to a non French national. In a more constructive role, they can also buy a farm in and then sell it on, the advantage to the purchaser being that it substantially reduces the hefty government taxes on land purchase. Finally they have a list of most agricultural properties for sale in the Hexagon. In this case the local officials at Auch were most helpful and I set out to inspect their list of possibles for Mr Mossman. Therefore when he returned a couple of weeks later, I was more than ready for him this time. It was Bastille Day and another scorcher, as The Sun would have said given the chance. After an abortive morning in the Landes the second farm just west of Vic Fenzansac seemed to appeal.

And so it came to pass that four months later and after protracted negotiations and several complications, I eventually sold my first farm and at the same time completed my first official sale in conjunction with *Donjon Immobilier*. The signings were usually long and complicated with the agent having to act as both interpreter and legal advisor for the client if he was English. The *notaires* were notionally neutral but didn't go out of their way to be helpful to the purchaser, hence the pressure on the agent. The agreed sale price I negotiated was just under two million francs, not a bad deal at all for the purchaser as it included in the price a substantial *maison de maître*, fifty seven hectares of irrigated arable land, five and half hectares of woodland and almost two hectares of vines. It was additionally very satisfactory for the vendor as he was both old and unwell and wanted to retire. It was also a cash purchase and the property had been on the market over two years. Yes, a very satisfactory deal all round. The overall commission at eight percent was exactly one hundred thousand francs which would have been very nice if it was all going to me. Unfortunately although I had done all the work I only received thirty five thousand francs. After I had deducted TVA or VAT my share had shrunk to under thirty thousand francs. Donjon received fifteen thousand francs for the privilege of providing me with my carte, my English colleague collected twenty five thousand francs for the taxing task of a single phone call and his fellow French agent in turn also received twenty five thousand francs for merely passing the client to him in the first place. If I was a bit younger I might have said it wasn't fair. Others might mention swings and roundabouts. *Mais c'est la vie, mon pauvre.* The deal was completed in November and was my only official one for the year. Then to add insult to injury the Département d' Impôt charged me pro rata TVA for the year for six times that amount. Yes, a good financial year all round.

Chapter 7 – The Nigerian Generals

It started with a fax in the middle of the night.

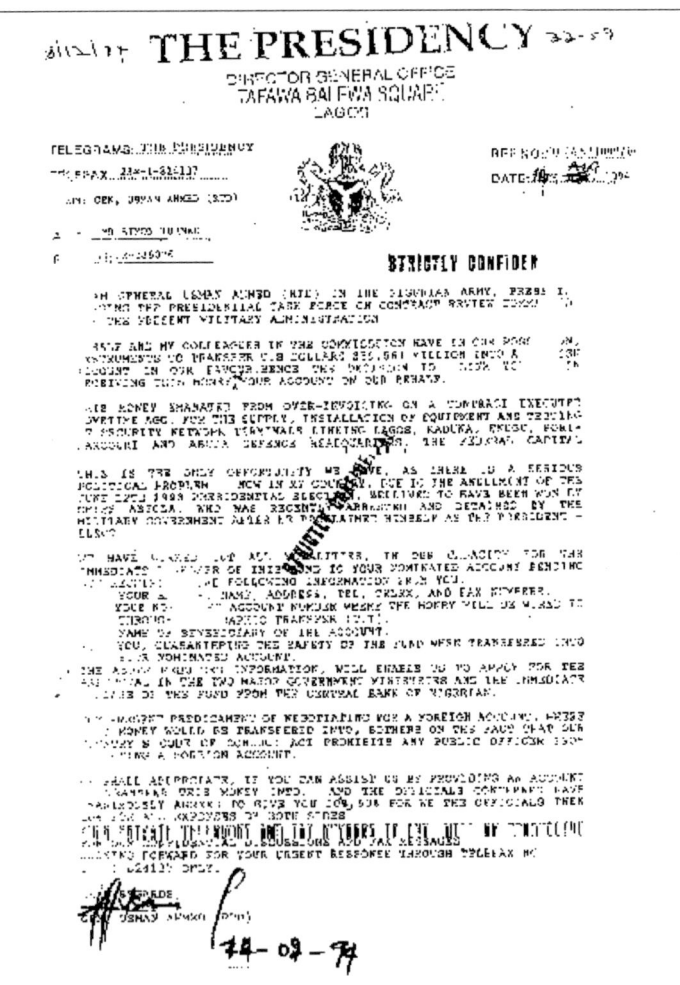

As the fax machine was in our bedroom cum study at *Heuré,* its chuntering woke me up with a start. Was I still dreaming? Was there really a benevolent God after all? More practically, what to do? It looked too good to be true. They say every man has his price and I had found mine, namely thirty nine point five six one million dollars. However I tried to pretend that I had not lost all my financial probity by replying coolly to The General on August 17th as follows:-

'With reference to your fax over the weekend, this matter may be of interest to me. However first I must explain I am a Real Estate Specialist, not a banker, and would only be too delighted to show you a number of top quality chateaux which could prove to be an excellent investment in the long term. However first I must know who recommended me and why choose my particular firm? Secondly I must have your assurance that I will not be acting outside the law in any way.'

Talk about wanting your cake and eating it. However after not getting a reply in the next five days I wrote again, not so coolly this time.

'On receipt of satisfactory reply to my fax sent over the weekend, I will be pleased to supply requested information immediately if you are still interested.'

Greed was getting the better of me. It was after I sent the second fax that I received the first of innumerable phone calls from Nigeria. The General's voice was deep, warm and trustworthy, but there again what did I know of such things? The General then sent me another fax a week later as follows:-

'Your fax messages of 17th 22nd inst, the subsequent telephone discussions and the inherent questionare therein, were well received and refer:

The recommendation and choice of your firm and person by a friend (Ishiaku Audu) as the best reference for this transaction was on the basis of the utililisation of my share of the fund on maturity and this above mentioned referee whose absolute admiration and interest is to favour your humility and most exceeding your sincere assistance to humanity irrespective of race, recommended too of your excellent accountability and probity in financial dealings. He further submitted that you have a unique equestrian property with historic manor house and forty (40) Acres Grassland, eight (8) Loose Boxes and useful Outbuildings at the rate of F. Fr 3.5M.

In view of the above and in consideration of the inherent property purchase I thought it wise to use your account for the passage of the said fund.

The transaction as far as am concern is very free from any encumbrances and would be executed within the ambit of all legal financial tenets applicable in the comity of nations. Therefore be reassured and hesitate no more in the supply of the requested information immediately.'

That was alright then, recommended by a guy I had never heard of to an illiterate Nigerian. But just to be on the safe side I had a word with Pierre Lagaillarde. Having carefully perused the faxes himself (his English was pretty good when it needed to be), Pierre was of the opinion that I was doing nothing illegal. If I had known then that he was a former revolutionary and had been both imprisoned and exiled, I think I would have been more sceptical of his definition of legality. I duly sent another fax to The General the next day as follows:-

'I would refer to your fax of 29th August, the contents of which have been carefully noted.

I regret that Mr Audu is not known to me personally but I accept in good faith the recommendation by a third party.

My usual commission on the completion of a real estate deal is 6% and I would be happy to accept the same figure in this particular transaction. I set out on page 2 my account number and other relevant details. I would stress that this is my personal account as it takes some time to open a new account. On receipt of the Bank Transfer I will open a new account for you with me as nominee. I will then transfer your money into this account (minus my six% commission) pending your further instructions.

I also personally guarantee the security of the fund after it has been transferred into my nominated account.

I hope that the above proposal is satisfactory, but should you require any further information please do not hesitate to contact me.'

I'm sure that the proposal was satisfactory to The General as he now had all my bank details. It was also very decent of me to work on 6 per cent commission only as opposed to the thirty per cent on offer.

After a further exchange of faxes everything appeared to be going swimmingly and I waited with bated breath for the arrival of the money. The General had assured me that the cheque was in the post. In fact I went into my bank in Fleurance every day for a week to check if my thirty nine and half million dollars had arrived safely in my account. I think we can safely say that I was delusional at the time. Funnily enough I am at this very moment fighting a case with the Inland Revenue where I am arguing that I was 'not of sound mind' and delusional when I signed a contract with them and it should be revoked. I think that the above proves that I have form on the subject.

I then received official faxed approval of the cheque from the Central Bank of Nigeria which I am very proud to display below. In fact the original fax has now been framed and occupies a prominent position on my office wall.

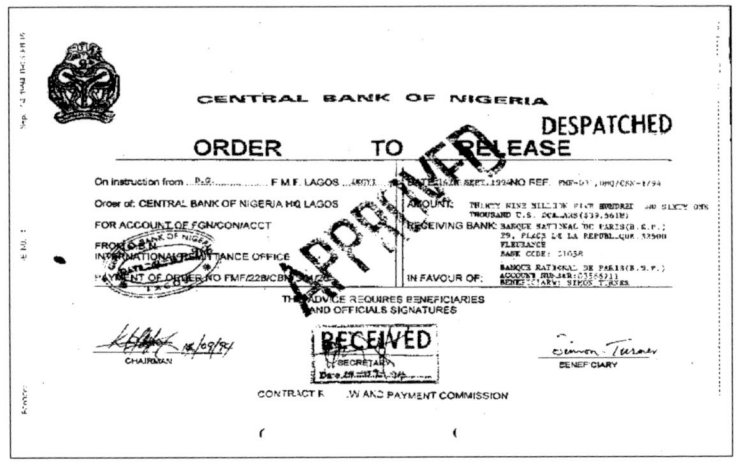

The sting was in the tail of course. At the same time I was being invited to first zip up to Paris to receive my Nigerian visa and then to nip over to Lagos with seventeen thousand two hundred dollars as 'the official signing fee' before the money would be released. What to do and what a to-do. I stalled and sent another fax to The General.

'I would refer to yesterday's faxes and telephone conversations and accordingly enclose a copy of the relevant page of my passport as promised.

However I am most concerned on two counts. First, in our original correspondence there was no mention that it would be necessary for me to come out to Lagos to finalize the arrangement. Secondly, neither in the original correspondence was I told that it would be necessary for me to raise the sum of $17,200. Why could not his sum be deducted directly from the Fund itself? In any event, to whom would the payment be payable?

I look forward to having your considered observations before I proceed any further.'

You bet I did.

The above fax got The General on the blower straightaway and he proceeded to show his other side. The oily charm had gone and the pressure was on. In desperation I had sent another fax:-

'With reference to yesterday's telephone conversations and earlier correspondence I am afraid I have bad news. I obviously have not got the equivalent of $17200 available in my own account but I had hoped to raise this sum by other means. Unfortunately all of these attempts have now proved abortive and I therefore regret that I will no longer be able to assist you in this matter.'

I thought that was the end but no, it only resulted in another menacing fax from The General:-

'I have been waiting for your call. I tried to reach you by phone. All my efforts proved abortive. Call me now as I am waiting'.'

By now I was shit scared and went to see Pierre Lagaillarde again. This time Pierre was right on the button and told me to get the hell out, although he expressed himself in rather more formal legal terms. I faxed back the next day:-

'I would refer to our recent telephone conversations and my faxes dated 16th and 17th September and would like to express forcibly the following two points.

1. I have no cash or credit available to me and all other avenues have been exhausted. This means that there is no chance whatsoever of me raising the extra $17200.

2. However more disturbing is that I have now received further legal advice which strongly advises me against proceeding any further with this matter. My lawyers are seriously worried about the legal implications and it would be very unwise of me to come to Nigeria.

Thus regretfully for the second time I must advise you that I don't see how I can be of further assistance to you, especially in the light of my remarks in paragraph 2.'

After that last fax I never heard from The General again. A narrow escape.

For those smug bastards who have read this chapter with increasing incredulity concerning my stupidity and gullibility, never underestimate the power of greed or desperation, or both. Also you must realize that back in August 1994, Advance –Fee Fraud or 419 Fraud as it has now come to be known had not been heard of outside Nigeria. The number '419' refers to the article of the Nigerian Criminal Code 'obtaining Property by false pretences'. Indeed the first prosecution of its kind was in the United States in October 1994 (only a few days after my narrow escape) where seven individuals were charged for conspiring to defraud the owner of a German computer software company out of more than $330,000. The indictment alleged that seven used interstate and international telephone wire communications in an elaborate scheme to defraud their target, Roland Woschny. The defendants made a series of telephone and facsimile contacts with Woschny in an effort to persuade him he was dealing with representatives of the Nigerian Government and the Central Bank of Nigeria. Between January and May 1994, these contacts allegedly led Woschny to believe he would receive about $22.3 million, described to him as money which was 'derived from an over-estimated contract with a Yugoslavian firm'. The money was allegedly to be paid to Woschny for his 'assistance and cooperation' in an alleged 'top secret project', and upon Woschny's payment of 'various expenses', amounting to $330,000.

Luckily for me, I had no money that could be stolen from my account, only a chunky overdraft which was no use at all to Nigerian swindlers.

The plausibility of the frauds at the time was reinforced by the fact that between 1993 and 1998 Nigeria was under the evil dictatorship of the late General Sani Abacha, and he and his gang that surrounded him are rumoured to have looted over $5 billion from its Central Bank in that time. Not that this country can be too proud of our contribution. British banks have only recently begun to repay Nigeria $1.3 billion of that loot that ended up in their hands. Obviously money laundering regulations weren't so tight in that era as is shown by the fact that Financial Services Authority investigated 23 banks identified by Nigerian authorities as receiving money and found 'significant control weaknesses'. Where oh where have I heard that wintry phrase recently? 'The file is now closed', said an FSA spokesman. That's alright then.

Of course Abacha's government was also guilty of innumerable human rights abuses including the notorious hanging of Ogoni activist and writer Ken Saro-Wiwa, after which Nigeria was immediately kicked out of the Commonwealth. Ken Saro-Wiwa was one of the truly great voices of conscience around the world and wrote the following inspiring words in a letter to International Pen just before his execution on November 10th 1995:-

'Whether I live or die is immaterial. It is enough to know that there are people who commit time, money and energy to fight this one evil (censorship) among so many others predominating worldwide. If they do not succeed today, they will succeed tomorrow. We keep on striving to make the world a better place for all of mankind. Each one contributing his bit, in his or her own way.

I salute you all.'

International Pen is a fine charity which is at the forefront of a laudable international movement aiming to promote literature, support the writing community and campaign for the rights and release of writers who have been unjustly imprisoned. English Pen is also currently waging a very powerful campaign for the wholesale reform of England's draconian libel laws. In an earlier letter to International Pen Saro-Wiwa wrote as follows:-

'I am delighted that literature led me to the realization that I had a specific responsibility for the Ogoni people as a part of the human race and that, using my pen, I could contribute towards the amelioration of the fate of an unfortunate people. I am happy to be a part of an organization like PEN which can put its intellectual and moral resources at the service of an otherwise unknown people. I am now convinced, more than ever, that the path of literature is the assured way to human salvation and to civilization. I hail the power of the pen.'

In his last work written in prison on about November 5th, 1995, just five days before his execution, and smuggled out to Pen, Saro-Wiwa chillingly foretells his own death.

'The familiar sound of the little drum woke me up. At the sight of the ghost, I laughed. Annoyed by my laughter, he dropped the drum and laid hold of his automatic weapon. He pointed it at me at close range. I did not flinch. He cocked the weapon and fingered the trigger. I did not bat an eyelid.

'Who are you?, I asked.

'I'm General Jeno Saidu.'

'Sounds like genocide to me,' I said.

'You should know.'

'What do you want?' I asked.

'I'm here to finish you,' replied he, in a gruff voice.

'General, stop swaggering. You do not impress me.'
'You will be impressed. I've finished all your Ogoni people
– men, women and children. Once I deal with you, my task
is done.'

'Go ahead,' I challenged him.

'You are not afraid to die?'

'No.'

'Why not?'

'I'm prepared to go with all my people whom you confess
to have murdered.'

'Yes I worked hard on them. I made short work of them.
All five hundred thousand of them. You are the last man.'

'So go ahead.'

'General Jeno Saidu, the ghost, shot into the ceiling. I
laughed.

'Why did you shoot into the ceiling and not into my chest?'

'You're still not afraid?'

'No, General.'

'And why not?'

'Because I have what is greater than your weapon.'
Whereupon, I said, after the English poet Blake.

'I will not cease from mental fight
Nor shall my pen sleep in my hand
Till we have built a new Ogoni
In Niger delta's pleasant land.'

Then I drew my pen from under the pillow. The General's
weapon fell from his hand and he slumped to his knees.....'

What a man. Unfortunately, Britain isn't very interested in
the ills of its former colonies these days. It much prefers to
invade Middle Eastern countries in which it has no interest
but oil. Well, Nigeria is the biggest producer of oil in Africa
but that fact doesn't seem to have registered with our
unenlightened rulers. Neither does the terrible pollution
caused by Shell-BP in the Niger delta. Oh, silly me, I had
forgotten that pollution doesn't matter in Africa.

With 606 oilfields, the Niger delta supplies 40% of all the
crude the United States imports and is the world capital of
oil pollution. Life expectancy in its rural communities, half
of which have no access to clean water, has fallen to little
more than forty over the last two generations. Locals
blame the oil that pollutes their land and can scarcely
believe the contrast with the steps taken by BP and the
United States government after the leak triggered by the
explosion that wrecked BP's Deepwater Horizon rig earlier
this year.

'If this Gulf incident had happened in Nigeria, neither the
government nor the company would have paid any
attention,' said the writer Ben Ikari, another member of the
benighted Ogoni people. 'This kind of spill happens all the
time in the delta. The oil companies just ignore it. The
lawmakers do not care and people must live with pollution
daily. The situation is now worse than it was thirty years
ago. Nothing is changing. When I see the efforts that are

being made in the United States I feel a great sense of sadness at the double standards. What they do in the United States and Europe is very different.'

'We see frantic efforts being made to stop the spill in the United States,' said Nnimo Bassey, Nigerian head of Friends of the Earth International. 'But in Nigeria, oil companies largely ignore their spills, cover them up and destroy people's livelihood and environments. The Gulf spill can be seen as a metaphor for what is happening daily in the oilfields of Nigeria and other parts of Africa. This has gone on for fifty years in Nigeria. People depend completely on the environment for their drinking water and farming and fishing. They are amazed that the President of the United States can be making speeches daily, because in Nigeria they would not hear a whimper. What we conclude from the Gulf of Mexico incident is that the oil companies are out of control. It is clear that BP has been blocking progressive legislation, both in the United States and here. They are now clearly a danger to the planet. The dangers of this happening again and again are high. They must be taken to the International Court of Justice.'

Is the International Court of Justice listening?

To return to the relatively trivial matter of fraud it was therefore quite possible that you could have been dealing with both members of the government and the Bank of Nigeria at one and the same time. Unfortunately for victims, Nigeria's efforts to fight the letter scams have been thoroughly inadequate. Amongst foreign observers, the overwhelming conviction was that the government was as corrupt as the crooks.

Abacha and his ruling clique thought otherwise. Amused and disbelieving observers woke up on April 1st the next year to learn that Abacha had just passed a new law called The Advanced Fee Fraud and Other Related Offenses Decree of 1995. But for several months after Abacha's law was announced, copies of the legislation were not available to lawyers, the public or even the special Fraud Unit, the elite police corps charged with combating the crime. 'It is clearly an April Fool's decree', remarked a local journalist at the time. It certainly wasn't a joke to Mr Woschny or other unfortunates who were conned.

What was a cracking joke, and the finest scam ever, was 'The Lost in Lagos Affair' in February 2009, involving the illustrious and Right Honourable Jack Straw, MP and ex-Justice Secretary to boot.

A message from Jack:-

'I misplaced my wallet on my way to the hotel where my money and other valuable things were kept...' 'I would like you to assist me with a soft loan urgently to settle my hotel bills and get myself back home.

It was an astonishing plea for help. A desperate Jack Straw, stranded in the steaming West African city of Lagos, with no money and nowhere to stay. His urgent demand: please send $3000 to bring me home. To alarmed members of the Blackburn Labour Party who received the email, it seemed strangely out of character for their globetrotting MP to be in sudden and urgent need of a cash bailout.

And so it was.

For Mr Straw, who during his tenure as Home Secretary pioneered a special unit to crack down on internet fraud, had become the latest victim to fall victim of an online scam.

Mr Straw's constituency Hotmail account was believed to be hacked into by what are thought by constituency workers to be Nigerian criminals who bombarded 200 contacts asking them to help the beleaguered minister. It claimed he had become separated from his pocket book while attending a summit called Empowering Youth to Fight Racism.

Some of Mr Straw's constituents seemed unmoved by his plight. One commented on the website of the Lancashire Telegraph, for which Mr Straw wrote a weekly column:-

'It's a shame Jack Straw was allegedly stranded in Nigeria as I cannot see many true Labour socialist workers who would have helped him out. Leave him in the heat.'

And so say all of us. Who knows, and miracles do happen, if Mr Straw stays out there long enough in the heat he may even do some good at last in that benighted country. He certainly has all the time in the world now.

Just to show 419 scams are still alive and well and living in West Africa, I recently received a most delightful email purportedly to have come from the Ivory Coast. That was the beauty of the old fax scams. At least they proved where the senders actually came from, even if you couldn't see the whites of their eyes so to speak:-

'Greetings

Please permit me to inform you of my desire of going into business relationship with you. I know my message will come to you as a surprise. Don't worry I was totally convinced to write you in reference of the transfer of my late father's money EU 5.9 million EUROS to your account for   onward   investment   (Real Estate/hospital/business/industries) in your,

I am MiSS LUCY KOFFI EDWARD the only daughter of the former Late General EDWARD KOFFI WALLAH OF Cote d'ivoire. My late Father was killed on 11th june 2003 following his role as a rebel leader against the government of Cote d'ivoire. Following this political crisis, I was forced to leave our village to Abidjan the capital city of Cote d'Ivoire for my life sake. My father deposited this said money in a prime bank here in Abidjan and used my name as the only daughter as the next of kin. And told me to seek for a foreign partner overseas that will help me for investment of this money into his or her country.

I got to know about this information and as well able to recover all the relevant documents regards to this deposit through his foreign adviser here in Abidjan. If you are truly disposed to assist me in transferring of this fund kindly, I am willing to offer you 15% of this money for your effort made during this transaction.write me through this email address. More information about the transferring of this money legally follows immediately after your positive reply. Awaiting your response soonest.

Best regards,

MISS LUCY KOFFI'

Thanks, but not tonight Lucy.

But I am very disappointed to report that purported friends of Lucy had better luck with the South Lanarkshire Council. Last autumn an allegedly African gang succeeded in conning the above mentioned cash-strapped council of £102000. Strathclyde Police are still investigating the fraud after South Lanarkshire admitted that an accounts worker had been taken in by the sting. The con involved a letter to the council where the writer claimed to be a real contractor and informed the local authority of a change in bank details and asking for its details in return. A council employee approved the change without checking and £102000 duly pinged out of the council's account and away into the fraudulent one, never to be seen or heard of again.

Because the crime was classed as an external fraud the council was not covered by the insurance. To rub salt into the wounds, the council was conned during the very week its own trading standards team were warning householders to be on their guard against a new council tax fraud. The fraud against the council was then discussed at a meeting of the Risk and Audit Scrutiny Forum. Yes really! And there was silly me thinking Forum was a rather rude men's magazine.

The chairman of this illustrious Forum was then reported as saying: 'The finance department was sent documents on letter headed paper to tell them to change bank details. It's not something I have ever seen before and it wasn't like an e-mail scam, which many people get sent to their home computers. We are not sure who has done this, but it has been professionally done by a gang in an African country.' If they are not sure who did it, how on earth can they blame an African gang? It seems rather unfair on Africans gangs to me.

Asked if someone should be sacked for the error the chairman said: 'If the person involved took all the appropriate action then they shouldn't be sacked. We will need to investigate if the person did follow the correct procedures.'

I would have thought that it would be far more worrying if the appropriately anonymous official <u>had</u> followed the correct procedures!

Chapter 8 Farms, Bailiffs and the European

January 95 and I had plenty of New Year's resolutions. One to work closer with M Rivière, two to 'Beat the Devil', namely depression, and three to further develop the SAFER link. Unfortunately I failed dismally on the first two counts because the third resolution should have provided me with the key to my financial salvation. Unwittingly I had stumbled on my true métier which was to act as a property search agent dealing almost exclusively in farms. As most of my clients were British and linguistically challenged, I naturally established a closer relationship with the prospective purchaser than the vendor. One exception was my old golfing pal Dennis. Early in March I had another interested customer for his ruined château. This time I managed to talk some sense into him, reiterating to him that if we didn't sell it this year there would be nothing left to sell as the roof had collapsed in the interim period since the last abortive sale and terminal decline was setting in. After the usual tough negotiations we had a sale at last and I was delighted with it having been involved so long with Dennis who was also struggling with his own cash flow problems. Yes, *une petite vente* but very rewarding personally. Not so rewarding was having to again hand over half of the commission to the same English client as in the Mossman affair, although in fairness to him he had managed two phone calls this time. It wasn't fair *comme d'habitude*.

Talking of cash flow problems the sale on Dennis' chateau wasn't finalized till the end of June which meant that I didn't earn even a single franc for the first six months of the year, except for a little fee I received for a newspaper article which we will come to in a minute. To temporarily ameliorate my finances during this period I did a fancy sidestep and sold the Corsa to some shady dealer who knew exactly what I was doing and naturally took maximum advantage. By some fluke the car was registered in my name so technically I could sell it, but of course what I was doing was highly illegal because of the express clause against doing so in my HP document. When the finance company found out some time later that I had sold their asset they naturally went ballistic and took immediate legal steps against me to get some of their money back.

Which brings me neatly on to another subject on which I do have unique knowledge, namely *huissières* or bailiffs. My specialist subject was limited to the two *huissières* of Fleurance and Lectoure. They were both ladies of a certain age but very different in looks and personality. The Lectoure one was a vivacious and pert brunette called Marie-Christine. Nicole of Fleurance was also very reasonable but did not have nearly such a good body as Marie-Christine. However her brother and deputy was a nasty bit of work. Much later I had one of my finest 'triumphs' on the last of his several attempts to repossess the Golf. This time the legal gods were with me. The brother hadn't done his homework as I still hadn't paid off the final instalment on this car either. However this time it was still registered with the finance company down as owner so when he turned up one sunny day with a malicious smile on his face and chewing a match to repossess the Golf it was with the greatest of pleasure that I told him in no uncertain French terms to fuck off. Then he realized he had cocked up big time and there was nothing he could do about it. Another brilliant Pyrrhic victory. I had several more run ins with him after that and he never forgave me for outsmarting him on that one occasion. Even in the depths of depression I still wasn't bad at the old French small print *de temps en temps*. But of course I had made another dangerous enemy, not a wise tactic at all in the long run.

Back on the agricultural stakes things were progressing. I had written to several English newspapers with suggested subjects for articles and eventually the not so mighty European took the bait and I was commissioned to write an article of a thousand words with a deadline of the same evening. I managed the feat just in the nick of time and was duly rewarded with a fee of one hundred pounds. The learned article came out under their nom de plume of Lawrence Begley, whoever he was when he was at home, and as The European is now of course defunct I don't need their kind permission to reproduce it below:

'There has been recent renewed interest in farms of all types reports Simon Turner specializing in agricultural properties from the Gers department west of Toulouse in South West France.

There is now strong European interest with English, Swiss, Dutch and especially German buyers, all keen to take advantage of the low values now prevailing in this delightful rural region also justly famous for its cuisine, foie gras and Armagnac. Arable land is now down to 15000 to 25000 Francs per hectare and progressively lower for pasture and upland resulting in some particularly interesting propositions on the market. I have a 50 hectare arable farm with good farmhouse and outbuildings at FF 1.35m, and a 71 hectare small country estate with maison de maitre, cottage and superb range of outbuildings where offers are invited in the region of FF3.25m.

The main crops are winter cereals, maize, sorghum, sunflowers, oil-seed rape, melons and garlic. In fact Saint Clar in the north east Gers and Beaumont-de-Lomagne in the Tarn and Garonne department are the twin garlic capitals of France. However sadly the future is looking bleak here for this ubiquitous crop with the price being savagely undercut by foreign imports, especially from the local bête noire, China. However prospects are much brighter for cereals, maize and oleaginous crops. Maize in fact produces the highest gross margins of all, with the vitally important proviso that the land is fully irrigable in this unforgiving climate. In fact up to some 30 years ago the Gers was mostly down to pasture until the construction of man-made lakes all round the region. However 'la sècheresse' (drought) of three years ago helped to ignite the decline for Gersois farmers. The Gers in fact is the biggest agricultural department in the whole of France being totally devoid of industry. Till recently land prices were touching 30.000 Francs per hectare and young local farmers borrowed heavily and indulged in new machinery in the delusion that the agricultural boom would continue. With the decline in prices in real terms, many have gone bankrupt with attendant problems for the local Credit Agricole bank, the main agricultural lender. Which brings me on to a key point. Good profits can be made but only by cash buyers not burdened by debt. Dennis, my golfing farmer friend says 'tout est fini' with his sons no longer following in his footsteps but heading for dynamic Toulouse with its high tech and concomitant Aerospatiale industries. Nevertheless, he agrees with my prognosis. Neither is there any local resentment to foreign buyers, with the average Gersois only too pleased to off-load their financial burdens and provide a 'patrimonie' (inheritance) for their offspring.

Buyers are split into three main categories: investors, 'hobby farmers' and professional farmers who all wish to take advantage of the depressed land values and simultaneously live in this most 'chaleureux' (literally warm or more accurately welcoming) backwater of rural France.

Of course with the first wave of predominantly English buyers of five years ago, many of those were seriously undercapitalized bringing about the attendant hard luck stories with which English papers and television seem to delight in publicizing. However today's buyer is much more hard nosed and prudent. They see a purchase as a primarily long term investment but which can also yield a satisfactory return on capital in the interim. One recent purchaser was a German industrial pharmacist who paid FF4.5m for 90 hectares of top quality irrigable land, the price including a delightful chateau and all material. He also has a farm in Germany and the land here is farmed by a local contractor. However the average German buyer, reports Karl Kossel, is buying around 40 hectares with good farmhouse for full time farming but introducing an element of tourism (i.e. camping and gites) and biological farming which is very much the rage. In fact Herr Kossel of H.K. Kossel and E. Stockbauer of Simorre has sold twenty farms in the last two years whilst the English have been procrastinating until recently.

To summarize, in my opinion farms are still an excellent investment in the northern sector of the Gers with its higher quality chalky/clay soil. In the south of the Gers which has more rugged terrain and woodland, I foresee an increasing trend to 'Green Tourism', leisure activities plus a continuing demand for horses, sheep and cattle. This historic area of Gascony had become increasingly moribund of late, but large infusions of capital from the above sources ate already revitalizing the region and enabling it to look confidently to the 21st century.

Simon Turner, a Chartered Surveyor and former restauranteur, can be located at Donjon Immobilier, Route de Toulouse, 32600, L'Isle Jourdain or telephone (33) 62-28-60-77.'

However this erudite and fascinating article didn't produce the hoped for riches. In fact the only two replies that I received were from one Chidi Ibeto at Africa Property Options Ltd who wanted to buy a 'stupendous' farm and a Dr Ahmed Talid who was apparently the chief accountant of the Nigerian Petroleum Corporation. However as the latter was only proposing to transfer thirty million dollars on this occasion I didn't bother to pursue the matter. Nor did I take up Mr Ibeto's kind but illiterate hope that 'this will mark the begginning of our business relationship'.

It seemed very appropriate that only fraudsters seemed to read 'Europe's First National Newspaper' as it was of course founded by that king of fraudsters, old Robert Maxwell himself, and The European well deserved the nickname given to it by Private Eye of 'Le Piss Pauvre'. It had been first published in May 1990 only a few months after the tearing down of the Berlin Wall and all the euphoria that went with the subsequent fall of the Iron Curtain. 'Captain Bob' thought he could convert that Europhoria by founding The European and utilizing it as a cheerleader for the ideal of a 'United States of Europe' which seemed a very real possibility at the time. He originally planned for a transnational newspaper to be printed in colour with articles in English, French and German. However as usual Maxwell's grandiose ideal proved impossible to realize and when it finally emerged in 1990, it had been scaled down to an English language weekly newspaper only. From the start Maxwell massaged the sales figures and when the first audited figures came out in February 1991 they were only 226,000, well below his promise to advertisers. The newspaper continued to decline and by the time of Maxwell's supposed suicide on November 5th, 1991, The European's London headquarters had been reduced to working a three day week. After Maxwell's death it was thought that the newspaper would fold completely but it was kept going long enough till after the New Year when the famously reclusive Barclay brothers became the new proprietors. Despite all the weighty money of the Barclay Brothers and later on in 1996 the equally weighty assistance of that old trooper Andrew Neil, 'Europe's National Newspaper' eventually folded in December, 1998, unlamented and unloved. The trouble was that the European suffered a debilitating schizophrenia from birth. It claimed to be a European newspaper published in English but it was viewed more as a British newspaper reporting on European affairs.

Maxwell's stated aim was to produce a newspaper for 'the housewife in Toulouse'. But the *Toulousain* housewife was already well catered for by her local version of *La Depèche* which catered for the whole of South West France. In addition, if Maxwell had done his homework he would have found out that, unlike the English, the French on the whole don't buy national newspapers.

That little history of The European above showed exactly why my article had fallen on such stony ground. Neither did it really cater for the property market despite its ambitions. I had found out the same fact the hard way in *The Independent* newspaper a few years earlier back in England. *The Independent* in those days was a cracking newspaper before it transmogrified into a tabloid, but it could never break the stranglehold that *The Times* and *Telegraph* exerted on the property advertising side.

I never did quite get the hang of this advertising lark as was shown by the fact that a tiny ad in the Farmers Weekly in England inserted about the same time as the above article produced two gems. One was a Danish farmer looking for a large farm with a sugar beet quota and a budget of ten million francs. The other was from an Irish entrepreneur who was also looking for a substantial enterprise, or to use his own inimitable terminology 'something rather tasty', to compliment his Pan European cattle running operations. A third very promising enquiry came out of the blue from the owner of a small Hampshire brewery who was looking for a quality vineyard with no specified budget which could provide both a nice little earner in his pub chain and an elegant holiday house into the bargain. Things were definitely looking up.

I started my research for my 'Great Dane' and found via SAFER that the prime sugar beet area was in North Eastern France but large units were apparently very thin on the ground. I also found some promising properties for Charley in central France near Poitiers plus a superb vineyard in the much underrated wine growing area of Buzet just north of Agen in the Lot and Garonne *department* for my brewery man. In these quests I was greatly helped by a multilingual Dutchman called Chris Vos who worked with the local SAFER at Auch. Chris became a good friend, although how good I wasn't to find out till after my return to England.

I also met plenty of other would be purchasers plus the usual *promeneurs*. One was a well known sculptor and his delightful wife but again I couldn't quite nail them down to actually sign on the dotted line. Another was a prominent Swiss scientist who somehow ended up buying in the Savoie region. I always seemed to end up befriending clients instead of actually selling them something. Would I now have more luck with 'The Big Three' in the New Year? *On verra.*

Chapter 9 - Death in Suffolk

Then in late May my brother phoned about Dad. He hadn't been well for a long time but David now thought that the situation was very grave indeed and very kindly paid for me to come over immediately as I of course had no funds for the flight. Therefore a week later I found myself very unexpectedly back in England. After staying a night with my brother in Surrey I took the opportunity of nipping down to Hampshire to see my vineyard client, Mr English, who was very pleasant if rather reticent, the shape of things to come. I then drove directly back to Suffolk to see my parents. I was very apprehensive about the reunion and with good reason. When I saw Dad I was shattered. His first words to me were devastating:-

'Do you still recognize me? I don't.'

And I didn't. My once oh so vigorous and distinguished looking father had been reduced to a wizened old man with a thin reedy voice. I stayed the weekend before I had to return to France but it was agonizing to see Dad just hobble about so feebly. He managed one last gigantic effort and joined Mum and me for lunch on my last day. When I shook his hand afterwards when he had retired back to his bed I whispered *au revoir* but I knew in my heart of hearts that I would never see him again. Two weeks later back in France I returned home to Heuré at lunchtime after some fruitless appointment where Mandy informed me that Mum had just phoned to say that Dad had died peacefully in his sleep the previous evening. I rushed off immediately for my next appointment in a daze and wept unashamedly for the first time in my adult memory.

Another two weeks later I was back in England again for Dad's non-religious Service of Remembrance. Dad had donated his body to Cambridge University for research so there wasn't that hideous coffin up front as there is for the usual Christian funeral. The service was held in an elegant recently restored eighteenth century former granary adjoining the River Stour, an edifice which was both structurally and spiritually eminently suitable. My brother spoke the opening words, my sister read the classic piece from Ecclesiastes, my four accomplished nieces played some music from Handel, long time neighbour Andrew Phillips spoke eloquently of his qualities and I wrapped up the proceedings by mangling a few nervous words from Wordsworth and Omar, Dad's own bible. It was very odd but it just struck me very forcibly at that precise moment that I could speak English so well if on normal form and French so badly even *en pleine forme*. What the hell was I doing with my life? My full text at the service was as follows:-

'Looking through some old papers the other day, I came across a letter Dad wrote to me about five years ago when he was recovering from major heart surgery which I think is rather appropriate on this occasion. I would like to quote from part of it:-

Thank you for your two letters, one cheerful and one not so cheerful. I too suffered a setback and a prolonged one at that, during and after I built up a firm resolve not to look backwards but to concentrate on today and the future. I had Edward Fitzgerald's Omar Khayyam with me as a P.O.W. and learnt by heart all seventy five verses, one of which I especially recall:-

The Moving Finger writes: and, having writ,
Moves on: nor all thy Piety nor Wit
Shall lure it back to cancel half a Line,
Nor all thy Tears wash out a Word of it .

So ends the first lesson of my philosophy to life!

And not a bad one at that.

Finally I would like to conclude with a few words from Tintern Abbey.

These beauteous forms,
Through a long absence, have not been to me
As a landscape to a blind man's eye:
But oft, in lonely rooms, and 'mid the din
Of towns and cities, I have owed to them,
In hours of weariness, sensations sweet,
Felt in the blood, and felt in the heart;
And passing even into my purer mind,
With tranquil restoration:- feelings too
Of unremembered pleasure; such perhaps,
As have no slight or trivial influence
On that best portion of a good person's life,
His little, nameless, unremembered, acts
Of kindness and of love.'

Dad's 'setback' referred to his four years with the Japanese after the fall of Singapore. He never spoke a word of his experiences but would never allow anything Japanese in the house. Normally he was very abstemious and the only occasion that I was aware of when he indulged in a glass of champagne was with fellow ex-prisoners of war to toast the death of Emperor Hirohito. However some years after his death we found out about a magnificent organization called Pacific Venture whereby grandchildren of ex POW's had fully paid trips to Hiroshima and other parts of Japan to see the other side of the coin as it were. All my three daughters were lucky enough to go and learn about the full horrors of war from the other side as well as meeting and developing friendships with young Japanese. Ironically in August 1995, just three months after Dad's death, Prime Minister Tomichi Murayama expressed for the first time the feeling of deep remorse and heartfelt apology for the tremendous damage and suffering caused by Japan's wartime action to the people of many countries. I am sure that Dad wouldn't have accepted the apology but thankfully it wasn't too late for his grandchildren. The previous year Prime Minister Murayama had paved the way for a ten year 100 billion yen Japanese 'Peace, Friendship and Exchange Initiative' to mark the fiftieth anniversary of the end of the Second World War in the Far East the following year. This initiative led to the foundation of Pacific Venture and I would now like to take the opportunity to thank in print the indefatigable Mrs Mary Grace Browning and Dr. R. John Pritchard for their magnificent efforts in this regard. Pacific Venture has gone from strength to strength over the years and the annual reunions gave the participants a continuing chance to share to each others progress through life while the receptions at the Japanese Embassy which my Daughter No 2 has been lucky to attend were magnificent affairs.

As I write this in December 2010, Pacific Venture has just had its last Grand Reunion as it was wound up after the last recent visit before Christmas, but that certainly doesn't invalidate any of the above. In fact it will leave an indelible memory on all those lucky participants which can only be beneficial to the peaceful aspirations of both countries.

After the service I met for the first time the person who now owned Dad's old estate agency business, a particularly poignant moment. I had often wondered if I would have made a worthy successor to Dad in the firm of H. J. Turner and Son if given the chance. Now I would never know.

With the kind permission of Alan Cocksedge I am pleased to reproduce his article from the East Anglian Times at the time.

GENTLEMAN HARRY DIES AT 78

A man who spent many years as a quietly effective benefactor for his town and campaigned on conservation issues has died.

Retired Chartered Surveyor Harry Turner helped found a Sudbury estate agency which for many years specialised in period properties.

While in business, Mr Turner, who was 78, refused to include photographs of his properties in adverts – choosing to rely on written descriptions. His gentlemanly, low-key sales pitch worked. By also advertising on a national scale, he was one of the first agents in East Anglia to capitalise on the gradually emerging post-war trend of weekenders, the retired and other people looking for properties on the Suffolk/Essex border.

During the war Mr Turner served with the Royal Artillery. He was captured by the Japanese at Singapore and worked on the infamous Burma railway.

Later he played for Sudbury Cricket Club and devoted many years to looking after the club's ground near his home.

He led a campaign to take over the Friars Meadow riverside area. He single-handedly – using his own mowers - proved to local authorities the rough grassland was suitable for recreation.

Part of his campaign also involved buying adjacent land and ensuring that it was transferred to public ownership at a peppercorn fee to provide part of the town's riverside walk.

Without him, the town's Quay Theatre would not have materialised. The one-time granary was due for demolition in the 1960's when he stepped in and converted it into an indoor cricket facility before making it available for Sudbury Dramatic Society.

In his retirement he purchased a site at Town Hill, Brent Eleigh and worked to reclaim the overgrown area. It will now be handed to the Suffolk Woodland Trust.

A humanist, Mr Turner has bequeathed his body for research at Cambridge University. No service will be held, but a meeting to commemorate his life will be arranged.

He leaves a widow, two children, a stepson and grandchildren.'

I must just add and correct a few points arising from Alan's very sympathetic piece. The Quay was in fact a former Victorian wharf and the granary was the adjoining building where we had Dad's service. In fact, Dad saved the former building with literally only hours to spare with a hastily arranged loan from the bank. Unlike me he always repaid his debts. The Theatre later won an award from the Royal Institution of Chartered Surveyors, but both their architectural reputations were severely tarnished by the carbuncle of a tatty old timber appendage. Shame on you both. Dad had done all the original structural work together with various contractors. Coming into the latter category was the demolition man who managed to hit a huge six of concrete out through the arrow like windows of the wharf into the old Scout Hut roof next to the Sudbury Rowing Club's head quarters. What a shot. The Scouts were apparently doing their Akela bit or whatever consenting Scouts do in private when the slab of concrete landed in their midst. Miraculously no-one was hurt. These days I think that the Health and Safety Police would probably have given Dad an ASBO.

After Dad had saved the wharf I freaked out when I heard that the Quay Theatre claimed all the credit for the restoration, carried out mostly with grant aid. Dad was too self-effacing to say even anything mildly critical, so I take this golden opportunity of reminding the people of Sudbury who they can really thank for the Quay Theatre building.

I must also correct Alan on another minor point. Dad 'sold' the Riverside Walk to the council for £1. If he had given it away he would have had to pay Capital Gains Tax. He had created that walk with his bare hands and his only mistake was that he hadn't retained the ownership of all the bat willows that he had planted in the 1950's which would have been worth several thousand pounds in today's market. But there again, he wasn't a mercenary bugger like myself, a point emphasised again when he bought and developed the old Congregational Church site in Friars Street for no personal profit whatsoever, despite some very tempting offers from local builders. It was originally thought that it would prove impossible to develop the site, but Dad found out the demarcation of every grave so they could all be avoided when construction eventually took place. Actually I am not mad on the Social Services building that resulted, although it has begun to nestle better into the plot with the mellowing of the years.

As Alan intimated above, Dad was also the unpaid groundsman for Sudbury Cricket Club for over twenty five years. He thought one of the finest compliments he was ever paid was when someone asked who that scruffy bugger in the old army shorts was and the answer was:-

'Oh, that's old Harry Turner the groundsman', not Mr Turner the estate agent note.

Very appropriate. Dad also did his level best for me as a father in his own way and I would like to repeat my own personal tribute:

On that best portion of a good man's life
His little, nameless, unremembered, acts
Of kindness and of love.

I then flew straight back to France to meet another sort of fate. A week later I happened to be reading P.D. James novel *Original Sin* when I came across the following passage:-

'There should, he thought, be a service designed for those without a religion. Probably there was and they could have discovered it if they had taken the trouble. It might be an interesting, and possibly even lucrative, publishing venture, a book of alternative funeral rites for humanists, atheists and agnostics, a formal ceremony of remembrance, a celebration of the human spirit with no reference to its possible continuing existence. Striding to the station, his long coat flapping open, he amused himself selecting passages of prose and verse which might be included. De la Mare's 'Look thy last on all things lovely, for a touch of nostalgic melancholy. Perhaps Oliver Gogarty's 'Non Dolet', Keats 'Ode to Autumn' if the dead person was old, and Shelley's 'To a Skylark' if he were young. Wordsworth's 'Lines written above Tintern Abbey' for the nature worshipper. There could be songs instead of hymns and the slow movement from Beethoven's 'Emperor Concerto' would be an appropriate funeral march. And there was, of course, always the third chapter of Ecclesiastes:

'To everything there is a season and a time to everyone under the heaven:
A time to be born, and a time to die; a time to plant, and a time to pluck up that which is planted;
A time to kill and a time to heal; a time to break down and a time to build up.'

And PD James was oh so right to conclude that 'these important rites of passage' were surely designed to comfort and minister to the needs of the living, since they could never touch the dead.

An extraordinary coincidence and a fitting conclusion.

Chapter 10 – The End

Back in France I had 'The Big Three' coming up. The first stop was my Great Dane. I had been plying him with properties since the beginning of the year and at last in September nailed him down to a visit. We eventually arranged a meeting only three days later at three in the afternoon at the small town of Houplines near Lille on the Belgium border in the extreme north east of France. The day before the meeting the agents phoned to say that they couldn't honour the appointment but my client had already left. Not a very promising start. The next morning at seven I caught the TGV from Agen. TGV, pronounced tay jay vay, was of course *Le Train à Grande Vitesse*. I had that usual disembodied feeling that came with anxiety. I just had to pull this one off. On the other hand I had always preferred outsiders. Not a feeble fiver each way on the favourite for me. Oh no, that would be far too mundane. Not so mundane were the incredible speeds we reached after Bordeaux without any sensation of speed save for the countryside flashing by in a blur. At eleven twenty two precisely the train pulled into Montparnasse Station in Paris dead on time. And dead is what I thought I was going to be half an hour later in the shitty bowels of the Metro where I sweated profusely during another vicious panic attack precipitated by claustrophobia. As I waited for the end all I could recall were those famous last words from Daphne du Maurier's chilling short story *Don't Look Now*:-

'What a bloody stupid way to die'.

Some time later I somehow found myself at the Gare du Nord and still in this world, but for better or for worse I wasn't quite sure.

However at the Gare du Nord my peace of mind wasn't exactly ameliorated by the overwhelming presence of heavily armed soldiers in the aftermath of the recent venomous Muslim terrorist attacks. It's funny that both Britain and America weren't too bothered about the Muslim threat till it happened on their own patches. I gulped down a couple of beers and caught the one o'clock TGV to Lille. Exactly an hour later we arrived in that fine city from where I got a taxi to Houplines. At ten to three I arrived outside the palatial premises of Cabinet Catteau. I was ten minutes early, *pas mal* after a journey of over one thousand kilometers. My Great Dane arrived precisely at three after a car journey of his own of over fifteen hundred kilometers. If clients are really serious they are always on time, *promeneurs* are always late. But first I had the task of explaining to a client whom I had never met before that the appointment was postponed till the morning. Luckily he took it well and I suggested we adjourn for a couple of *petits cafés* and go more thoroughly through his situation. Apparently he wanted to move lock, stock and barrel from his large farm in Denmark and set up in France where the land was a lot cheaper. And he was obsessed with sugarbeet (*betteraves*) and sugar beet quotas. However by now I was a regular subscriber to France Agricole and shit hot on yields, crops and shit in general. We then checked into a local hostelry where my wealthy client booked us both in at a modest four hundred and fifty francs a night, breakfast extra. Of course two of my biggest of an increasing litany of calamitous errors was first in not having a *mandat de récherche* signed in advance and second not getting an advance on expenses. Would my new credit card stand the strain?

The next morning we met Monsieur Catteau junior and I have to say that in all my ill begone property days Jean-Michel Catteau was the most arrogant agent I have ever met. He made Messrs Bidwells and Strutt and Parker look like mere amateurs. He certainly had blond youthful charm, a blood red Porsche and was annoyingly good looking into the bargain, but I wasn't jealous. His disdain for us both was breathtaking, but after lecturing us on the shortage of farms in the ten million franc range and various methods of tax evasion schemes, he passed us dismissively off to his lackey, Monsieur Macaigne. GD had brought his Saab and we now proceeded to whizz round a large portion of north eastern France at great speed. First stop was only fifty kilometres south of Houplines in a very flat area with a smelly factory on one side and an interesting array of pylons on the other. It was certainly very conveniently situated, but not what GD had in mind. The next pit stop was another hundred k's south down the *autoroute* before we turned off into delightfully undulating deer country in the little known Aisne department near Soissons. This farm was a lot better but with an extremely modest farm house. By this time it was getting late and GD surpassed himself by finding a super international complex at a cheeky price of seven hundred francs bed and brek. Naturally I didn't sleep very well and the next morning before breakfast had another scary panic attack. Would I survive the pace? Would I survive at all?

After breakfast it was quickly on past Reims, Éparnay and rolling champagne country where the fields were monumental in size and made East Anglia look like an ultra mini granary. Further south still we came to the '*très belle*' unit cunningly severed by the motorway which M Catteau had conveniently forgotten to mention. After that I had planned to show GD an excellent sounding farm south of Paris that I had found through SAFER. In fact it sounded by far the most promising proposition of the lot. But GD was adamant that he preferred the north east area and went funny on me. He took me into Troyes and dumped me peremptorily at the railway station saying he would be in touch. One moment we were in deep, friendly conversation and the next he had totally gone. Thank heavens for little clients, without them what would little agents do.

So there I was, bemused of Troyes, and I will leave you to work out how to pronounce that ancient tip. I had just missed the Paris train by a matter of minutes and the next one wasn't due for another three hours, an unhappy foretaste of things to come. After three hours of Troyes I had seen quite enough thank you, and to cut a long story short Mandy eventually picked up an exhausted *agent immobilier* from Montauban station at midnight. One down, two to go.

Next came Mr English who was again meticulously punctual despite a long car journey from the Languedoc wine area. He got a free case of Buzet but seemed far more interested in a property specializing in white wine as well. However I had now grasped his obsession with Nick Ryman and the Bergerac region and promised to see what I could find in another underrated sector. It adjoins the vast Bordeaux appellation region which although the latter of course includes some of the finest wines in the world it also includes a staggering percentage of mediocrity. For those who don't know the story, Nick Ryman became a multi-millionaire when he sold the Ryman family stationery in 1973. He then tried to live his own dream of owning a chateau and vineyard in France. He found and fell in love with the beautiful Château de la Jaubertie in the Dordogne near Brive. He went on to make some of the finest wines in the Bergerac area, together with the later, acrimonious help of his son Hugh, a fine winemaker in his own right. To those of you who are interested, Jeremy Josephs has written a fascinating book called 'A Château in the Dordogne' about the trials and tribulations of the Ryman family in the pursuit of their dream to beat the French at their own game. Hugh Ryman was later to set up on his own account before becoming one of the very first flying wine makers. I think Mr English wanted to emulate Nick Ryman in producing top quality wines in the Bergerac area, but without the family aggravation.

Bringing up the rear was Charley H. I had had many interesting conversations with him during the course of the year but he could never seem to make it outside his native Ireland. Finally in October he shocked me by actually venturing across the water. We agreed to meet in the small village of Bellac between Limoges and Poitiers. In the next few months I was to become an expert on the French railway system and individual provincial stations. Oh yes, I was an expert on every subject except for my supposed specialist subject. The *Gare des Bénédictins* at Limoges is an impressive copper domed thirties effort and even has a romantic name into the bargain. Liverpool Street just doesn't have the same ring, does it? Or Saint Pancreas or Paddington Bear. The *Gare de Poitiers* is a cheerfully modern pastiche, while the *Gare de Bordeax-Saint Jean* is splendidly late Victorian with a magnificent roof designed by Gustave Eiffel of Eiffel Tower fame. Last but by no means least comes the *Gare d'Agen*. This station is not only structurally elegant but the café provides a lively meeting place for the young, as well as having a restaurant recommended by none other than Rick Stein. Contrast the glass Nissen hut which professes to be Colchester station. The latter station on a foggy November day must be England's nearest equivalent to a Gulag. Come on Network Rail, do something.

I had gone up by train to Bellac because Mandy needed the Golf, although if the truth be known I thought the latter a bit humble for the obviously wealthy entrepreneur that I was about to meet. I hadn't been so caring on a few other occasions when she had been left to walk six kilometers across country to work in Saint Clar! I cruised up to Limoges and after two hours of coffeeing at the station, had a lovely little trip through the woods on a tiny branch line train. An enchanting journey and a welcome break from reality. At Bellac I struggled with my case to the local hotel which was some distance from the station. There I was informed that my client had just arrived. He was much younger than I expected, mid thirties I suppose, very affable but piercingly watchful. I had banked on him hiring a car and when I had found out that he had come all the way by public transport as well, was forced to offer a very lame explanation for the absence of mine. Luckily I got hold of the local agent Monsieur de la Pôterie who arranged to pick us up in the morning in his own car. The next morning the suave MP turned up in a not so suave 2CV. What a start. Charley dominated the front of the car with MP whilst I lurked in the back with his bloody great labrador dog. What a *cauchemar* (nightmare). The first two farms weren't of much interest but the third one was distinctly promising, except for the giant disused quarry at the entrance and more huge pylons totally ruining the outlook of the extravagantly restored chateau. However there was the little matter of two hundred hectares of prime pasture and woodlands at a tasty asking price of seven million francs. Four or five per cent of that didn't seem too bad, or even two and a half if it came to the worst. However not so precipitate, *mon petit*. Charley wasn't to be rushed into anything except to hire a car from Poitiers that evening which meant that MP having to do an extra two hundred kilometer round trip which he obviously wasn't very keen on. He certainly didn't want to work too hard to earn his vast commissions and he certainly couldn't work on Sundays, where he was involved in the traditional twin pastimes of la chasse and le déjeuner. *Pas de discussion.* Anyway Charley and I shuffled about ineffectively on Sunday morning before retiring hurt to the station at Poitiers. As was to become an annoyingly typical occurrence he had a train leaving for Paris in five minutes while I had another three hour wait again for mine down south. I know Poitiers has its architectural delights but I wasn't very interested on that Sunday afternoon so I sat in the sun and had a few beers. I eventually got back to Agen station late in the evening dispirited and buggered. Two 'total immersion' days with a client is hard work and I had got absolutely nothing to show for my pains. The 'Big Three' had disappeared into the sunset.

After all these setbacks came a pleasant surprise. I had been corresponding with a Cumbrian farmer for over eighteen months before he suddenly phoned me out of the blue and said he had now sold his farm and was ready to go. A couple of farm details in the Vienne department that I had originally got for Charley appealed to him. We therefore arranged to meet at the little town of Confolens in the Haute Vienne department.

Here I must give a little background on the local agent we were going to see. We had got on very well on the phone at first until I mentioned shared commission. JR turned out to be a Glaswegian mugger impersonating as an *agent immobilier* as he quoted me the rate appropriate to an agent working from England. Instead of discussing it with M Rivière or getting my client to sign a *mandat de recherche*, as usual I took the soft option of agreeing with him for the time being and hoping to sort things out later, just like my whole policy in life in fact. JR didn't exactly ingratiate himself with me further by being over half an hour late for the first appointment although he only lived on the doorstep whilst my client and I had driven vast distances to be there on time. Anyway I bit my tongue as he took us round and in fairness to him he showed an excellent grasp of local agricultural matters and a fluent if guttural command of the French language. We saw a few farms before my client, Mr Cooke, returned to England to report to his wife.

Back home I thought about the possibilities. Mr Cooke wanted a good grassland farm and this obviously ruled out the hot, arable wasteland of the south west. I therefore craftily tried to distract him away from the Confolens area to the Nevers region to the east where I had found some strong possibilities via the local SAFER. This meant yet another long trip up north in the Golf through Limoges and my bogey town, Argentan-sur-Creuse. It also meant Mandy was without transport so she had to get out her willies again to set off and walk to Saint Clar in the rain. I had assured her the night before that I'd deliver the goods this time. 'It will be worth it', I'd idly and boastfully promised. In fact I was more apprehensive about repeating my route of that ill-fated day over six years earlier. However this time I took the short cut directly to Cahors where the fiercesome old N20 had partly been upgraded to an autoroute which greatly ameliorated my journey. That day I faced the fucking fear and beat it hands down and even had a coffee in Argentan to celebrate. *Bravo.* But I hadn't faced Mandy with the truth which was an even tougher task. From there I drove on to Saint Armand-Montrond in the Cher department where I met up with Mr Cooke and his wife. Again Mr Cooke hadn't lived up to his telephone manner being twenty years older than my expectations but he was bluff, avuncular and very easy going. His wife was much younger and frighteningly naive of France in general, appearing a lost soul from the frozen north. After visiting the first farm on my list which proved to be disappointing it was on to Nevers. The latter is a hill town spectacularly perched above the banks of the River Loire, with the not so spectacular racing circuit of Magny Cours a few k's away. We met up with the local SAFER agency where we were assigned a young but very knowledgeable officer to show us around. We were in prime Charolais beef country with lush green fields, rolling countryside, large tracts of broadleafed woodland and *pas un Anglais* in sight. Not surprising really as the east wind cut through us like a knife and Mr Cooke thought it was too much like home, not what he had in mind at all. Reluctantly I travelled back a couple of hundred kilometres west to JR country, where I left Mr Cooke to open negotiations on the original farm he had seen, which co-incidentally was also in a commune called Isle Jourdain. I then returned home as I thought he had enough of my endless feuding with JR by then, but guided him by fax and phone through the *compromise de vente* after they had agreed a price.

In the interim I had also discovered France's newest nuclear power station being built down the road on the River Vienne but Mr Cooke seemed unfazed about this newest installation in France having lived for many years within melt down distance of the antiquated monstrosity of Windscale cum Sellafield in England. In fact he seemed unfazed by anything at all being the proverbially laid back Lancastrian. However the fact that I was not there for the actual signing enabled JR to totally outwit me by getting him to sign a *mandat de recherche* direct with Nowak Immobilier, his own office. The sale price was almost identical to the Mossman sale I had arranged in the Gers but Charentais rates pushed up the total commission this time by fifty per cent to a whopping one hundred and fifty thousand francs. All this time JR had continued to outwit me on the commission front and ended negotiations with the following dismissive fax to me.

'Thank you for your fax 15th re Cooke. I trust he'll find something to suit him on this trip.

Re your comments on the subject of commission. We work on the same basis with all external agents be they be based in France or any other country and trust that all these agents follow up on their clients with a full service. We also never favour one property or another depending on the amount of money we can get from it. We always try to act in the best interests of our client.

The question of commission is NOT open to debate and the thought of Mr Nowak PERSONALLY sending out details is quite amusing. He has two secretaries to do that. Your request was in fact dealt with by one of them and until I had suggested it there was no question of you receiving ANY COMMISSION at all.

If you wish to work with us please confirm by fax. If not, as I have said, I'm sure you'll find another agent in the area to suit your needs, bearing in mind that none of them sell even a tenth of the amount we sell.'

What breathtaking arrogance but I had to bite the bullet and would receive a mere thirty thousand francs for all my troubles despite M Rivière calling Nowak a bandit. In turn JR told Mr Cooke that M. Rivière was sabotaging the deal. Mr Cooke was naturally furious and called him 'a bloody man and a liar'. What a mess. In the end I had to drive all the way up north again for the *Acte Définitive* in late January where the condescending *notaire* made me feel very small while JR kept my client well away from me. It was a very lonely long drive back that cold winter's afternoon.

The previous week before my trip up to Civray had brutally brought home the parlous state of my finances when I was stopped near Saint Clar by the local gendarmerie during a random sweep. The young gendarme was another old adversary who was delighted to arrest me for the hideous French crimes of no road fund tax or insurance, and then took me back to the police station where he impounded my car. I thought for the umpteenth time that this was it, but again somebody must have been keeping some sort of weather eye out for me as the chef of the police station was none other than the father of one of Daughter No 1's school friends. He very benevolently allowed me to go home with my car and obtain the road fund licence within twenty four hours, much to the chagrin of the young gendarme, having previously verified with my insurance company that I was still covered even though I hadn't yet paid for the renewal.

My relatively meagre share of the proceeds from the Cooke sale at least enabled me to fight another day. Mr English came and went again as I plied him with possibilities. I thought I had finally cracked it with him by finding an excellent vineyard very near the town of Bergerac itself which produced both red and white wine as he required, but tantalizingly the house wasn't quite good enough. I found out much later that Mr English eventually purchased a very fine property indeed, the Château de Fayolle at Saussignac south west of Bergerac. It has subsequently been sympathetically restored to a very high standard and is now available to rent for those with deep pockets. It is also licensed to hold marriage ceremonies in the lovely old chapel in the grounds. In fact, a perfect place to hold a fairy-tale wedding.

After Mr English's departure the Great Dane finally disappeared up his own *betteraves* but back came reliable old Charley. Off I went to Poitiers again by train and endured another two hour wait at the station. Christ, I knew every mock pillar by now as I gazed back at it from my adopted café. The waitress had a see-through blouse, good breasts but no welcoming smile. She probably thought I was a sad old voyeur and she was probably right. Along came Charley at last, charming as ever and with mobile phone in hand as ever. The latter phenomenon hadn't caught on yet in France, and the coverage in the south was so poor that I eventually decided not to pay my exorbitant *factures (bills)*. On the previous occasion Charley had managed to hire a very acceptable Renault Mégane but this time he could only get hold of a poky Clio. First we drove a hundred kilometers east to a property near Châteauroux where we found another SAFER dud. Then off we whizzed down south beyond Limoges where we eventually found a singularly grotty hotel. The next day we went further south still to Bergerac where we saw another possibility, but unfortunately the access roads apparently weren't good enough for Charley's jumbo lorries. On to Agen where we had a long delay whilst sorted out a problem with one of his lorry drivers at Barcelona. Finally it was back to the Gers and a quick snack at Fleurance where I abandoned Charley for the night. I was totally knackered by the time I got back to Heuré as well as being half blinded by a missing contact lens. Not a good day at the office.

The next day we met up with Chris Vos again south of Auch near Mirande and saw his 'Pearl of Gascony' farm but Charley was proving very difficult to please, so off we raced to the lovely Ariège area where we saw a delightful property with truly fantastic views of the Pyrenees. However Charley was still thinking only in punt signs and like the Gascons, was of the opinion that views don't pay the bills. It was another stinking hot day but we then set off again at four in the afternoon on a three hundred kilometre trip back up to Angoulème in the Charente *département* in the piddling little Clio with no air conditioning, and we were both sweating and knackered by nine o'clock at journey's end where we found an excellent family hotel in La Rochefoucald quaintly named *La Vieille Auberge de la Carpe d'Or*. The next morning I saw a glimmer of hope at another farm with MP near to where Mr Cooke had bought. The trouble was that JR had first sent me the details before SAFER so there would be a nice clash of interests if I ever clinched a sale. Then it was back to Poitiers station where Charley zoomed off to Paris *tout de suite* while I had my usual two hour wait.

When Charley returned in July this was positively my final, final chance. In fact I had to borrow five thousand francs from M Rivière to enable me to make the trip. By the way Monsieur R, your cheque is now in the post. During all this time I was still playing golf furiously whilst closing my mind to the world outside, including Mandy and the girls. I was no longer there mentally. All I could hear was Test Match Special on the radio and all I could manage was literary escapism accompanied by more liquid escapism.

Back to Poitiers station. God, I hated the place by now. Charley had just taken his children to Futuroscope and afterwards we adjourned appropriately to a Macdonalds to assuage his 'difficult' kids. By contrast his wife was delightful, elegant and charming, a true Irish belle. Then straightaway to the farm near Confolens in a Renault Espace which Charley had sensibly hired in advance this time. I had noticed on previous occasions that Charley was a rather reckless driver on rough farm roads, but mindful that he was the client and he was doing the hiring I kept my mouth firmly shut. However on this occasion after one spectacular bump on the sump, his son quietly asked Dad what was the big black trail following him. Of course he had only gone and smashed the bloody thing completely. After an uncomfortable four hour wait for reinforcements we set off in Renault Espace *numero deux* back to the Dordogne where Charley soon found a lovely hotel in a lovely setting called the Hostellerie Saint Jacques in the small village of Saint-Saud En Périgord. If I had been on a romantic weekend with Mandy it would have been perfect, but Donjon's cheque had only covered my overdraft so it meant I would have to present a cheque *'en bois'* in the morning. *En bois* literally means in wood, come to think of it a very good description, but of course really means a cheque presented without funds or to bounce a cheque. This was strictly illegal in France but I was past caring by now as we sat down to a sumptuous meal that evening. The Dordogne property the next day was another Pôterie damp squid. God, he had a mega attitude problem. Back north we trailed and pitched up in a glorious setting adjoining the River Vienne where we stayed at some seriously expensive Nissen huts which were masquerading as the Hôtel Grand de Vienne. Ironically the owners were English but I had to be fair so I presented them with another *chèque on bois* in the morning as well. I know Robert Maxwell was nicknamed 'The Bouncing Czec' but I was now the undisputed 'Bouncer of Cheques'. After another gourmet's delight at the Michelin listed La Grimolée restaurant adjacent to the hotel, I made my last fatal sally. It was the Charge of the Light Brigade all over again. Over numerous armagnacs and fags far into the night, I informed the normally abstemious Mrs CH that she would be totally unsuited to living in this rough and ready part of France, surely my finest hour as an estate agent.

After that it was naturally downhill all the way back to Poitiers station for the last time. I said my farewells to Charley and to the *immobilier* world for good. I have often wondered since if he ever did buy a property in France. At the time of course I didn't wonder or care at all. I limped home to Heuré and waited for the end.

'Now the sun's gone to hell
And the moon's riding high
Let me bid you farewell
Every man has to die.'

Chapter 11 – Retreat to England

I was awakened from my reverie by the sounds of laughter as the others relaxed in the remnants of a sad Gascon sunset. However I was only there in body, not in spirit. Another glass of red wine? *Pourquoi pas*? That's better. Let's drink to oblivion. *Ā votre santé.*

Later that evening Mandy said in desperation that we had to do something. Anything. Eventually she came up with a sort of solution, even if it didn't look exactly like salvation to me. By chance we had some very old friends from England staying with us at the time, and unbeknown to me, they decided with Mandy to take me back to England with them. The next day duly found me duly packed up and slumped in the back of D and A's old Peugeot Estate heading north for England after seven years of financial famine and mental torment in France. Was it too late to repair the damage? *On verra.*

I travelled back to England in a total daze. I smelt no sea and saw no sky. I looked into the void and what did I see? Absolute zero. The darkness in my soul obliterated all light. The only thing visible to my bloodshot eyes was debt, debt and more damned debt, dragging me down to the depths of despair. Where had it all gone wrong? I had been born with a silver spoon in my big ugly mouth, but my Anglo Saxon hubris had long ago disintegrated into a Gallic nemesis. Abject and total failure. There was no future, only a pathetic past. My addled brain worked out with some convoluted logic the simple fact that I was worth plus one hundred and fifty thousand pounds dead but minus twenty five thousand pounds alive. Contrary to popular opinion and various writers of detective novels suicide doesn't always invalidate a life insurance policy.

With my Equitable Life policy it was only specifically excluded during the first year of the contract which was now some fifteen years ago. But of course as I have told you before ad nauseam I was bloody good at the small print when it suited me. However the truth was that I was utterly worthless either way so what the hell.

'What is hell
Hell is oneself
Hell is alone...'

But I hadn't even got the guts to confront it right there and then. God had called my bluff. It didn't really matter. It was all so pointless. I was going down, down, down.......

Back in England I spent a few days at D and A's watching another English debacle in the final Test Match at the Oval against Pakistan and also did some desultory long distance solitary walking. After a few days I was eventually persuaded by the rest of the family to make contact with my mother and she invited me to stay with her in Sudbury 'for the time being'. Ironically, we met up in Great Dunmow, the scene of my earlier demise.

What the hell was I suddenly doing in Silly Suffolk again staying with my elderly mother? I was a forty seven year old married man with three children, for Christ's sake, not a middle-aged bachelor with an Oedipus complex. *Pas de problème*. Depression and mental illness didn't exist in the Turner psyche and even if they did, you certainly didn't talk about it. That's dirty talk, far worse than sexual peccadilloes. However the Turner family in all its wisdom seemed to think that my salvation lay in the good old Protestant work ethic. Was I willing and able to work? Yes, and no. A big no to apple picking. Yes perhaps to looking for a job on the property scene again. So began a fruitless two month search, starting by trying to get reinstated back in the Valuation Office, but they sensibly declined my application. I then got an interview with a well known national firm of estate agents, Messrs Abbots if you really want to know, where their two hatchet men destroyed me on the touchy subject of my apparent inability to get on with people. However what made it worse was that I knew in my heart of hearts they were dead right because I was no team member. Bugger male bonding. Pass on female bonding.

My solution was simplicity itself. If no one wished to employ me I would employ myself. I still had to beat my father. From the grave his achievements were still my obsession; and nemesis. For the time being I was vaguely self-sufficient as I was now registered on the dole. I knew my mother thought this wrong in principle, especially as I had been out of the country for seven long years. I should be made to pay for my transgressions. How about seven years hard labour in a factory instead? And how could I afford to drink and smoke? What she just didn't grasp was the fact that an addict doesn't need to be able to afford it but must have his fix at any cost to himself. Chorus from Omar:

Ah, my Beloved, fill the cup that clears
TO-DAY of past Regrets and future Fears.

No cheer there.

I therefore enrolled on two courses at Otley College near Ipswich, one in computing and the other in a so-called Owner Management course. Me, who couldn't even switch on a computer let alone tell you what a floppy disc was or define a megabyte except hesitantly suggest that it was some sort of Jumbo Macdonalds. Property search was getting big in England and I naively thought I could do streets better this time round on home territory and with a proper battle plan. It was now into a very murky November and it looked like we had a buyer for Heuré and there was a possibility that the family could be back for Christmas. Mum had paid off my biggest debts in France to get the banks off my back and front and Mandy had managed to clear the bounced cheques I had incurred during my last sally with Charley H plus the T Zoid driver I had inexplicably 'purchased' for fifteen hundred francs in June. How could a man who was totally broke go ahead and buy the latest golf club? He must have been totally insane. I rest my case.

Of course I was now disbarred from holding a bank account in France for ten years so that was the end of my French business career. *Tant pis*. Otherwise things were apparently looking up as I pressed ahead with the notion that I could be the finest property search agent in Suffolk. Depression intertwined with hubris was a dangerous cocktail. However for the time being my mental state was stuck rigidly in neutral whilst I did my courses in a trance and cut myself off totally from the outside world. I didn't want to see any other live people if possible and I certainly didn't wish to relive those 'Glory Days' back at the rugby club. I was a failure not for display.

Come December and more setbacks. Our house sale fell through and the family was destined to remain in France for the indefinite future. I had almost finished the Otley courses and was ready to start my own property search business as Turners as the name was still worth quite a lot of goodwill in my estimation. That's when I hit the wall. My mother didn't want me to use my own birthright. She would feel 'uncomfortable' about it. Dad had not only given away the business for the proverbial song but I wouldn't be allowed either to utilize the family name. She probably didn't want me to besmirch his hallowed memory. I was incandescent with anger, anger that was still smouldering inside me when I hit the Toulousain tarmac two weeks later for a Christmas family reunion. Some reunion. I harangued Mandy all the way back to Heuré from the airport about some imagined indignities that had befallen me and arrived completely oblivious of the show the girls had put on specially for my benefit or the fact that they had totally redecorated the house. I then got pissed after everyone had gone to bed.

'Oh, as I watched him on the stage
My hands were filled with fists of rage.
No angel born in hell
Could break that satan's spell.
And as the flames climbed into the night
To light the sacrificial rite,
I saw satan laughing with delight
The day the music died.'

Mandy was disgusted, despairing and dismayed all at the same time. She had been led to believe by the family that I was much better. After an icy week I then tried to irrevocably break the fragile remnants of our marriage by just walking away from her at Toulouse Airport without a word of goodbye or even so much as a semblance of a backward glance. Luckily I had retained the tiniest semblance of sanity in that battered pea brain and muttered a little aside to my sister when she picked me up from the airport in England that I had really blown it this time. Appropriately, it was now Boxing Day. She then phoned Mandy and managed to salvage a toe hold so that I could cling to the wreckage of a marriage for a while longer. I have always been a trifle hard on my sister so I suppose I should give her a little belated thank you now. Thanks sis.

Back 'home' in Suffolk with no house sale on the horizon and with zero capital to set up my business, the banks were naturally reluctant to push any more pounds my way despite my impressive business plan. Mandy on the other hand had turned to the French authorities who happily continued to give her support for the children since they were doing well at school and she was actually working, albeit for a modest salary teaching English.

Back to her ne'er-do-well husband who still had his head firmly in the clouds. However, the banks had turned me down flat for totally the wrong reasons. The plan itself was flawless but they wouldn't even look at it. What they should have done instead was to look inside my head and then turned me down. A plea to banks. A little less emphasis on figures and a little more on psychology.

Next I had more bad news. I heard that the new Benefits Agency had cut off my income support. It had been necessary to sign off to leave the country, even though it was for only a week over the Christmas period. However unknown to me since I first signed on in September, the Conservative government had brought in a new Jobseekers Allowance scheme in another cynical attempt to manipulate the unemployment figures. Sound familiar? After six weeks of fruitless correspondence I am delighted to set out below the Benefits Agency's final written decision which was such an inspired piece of perverted logic that I am proud to reproduce it in full. Of course I wasn't so delighted at the time.

'Dear Sir

Thank you for your telephone call of 4/3/97 concerning the legislation used to decide your claim to the Jobseekers Allowance.

Decisions are made by considering the relevant Act. In this case, the Jobseekers Act 1995. The act gives the basic intention to the law.

In order to apply these principles, we use statutory instruments – in this case the JSA Regulations 1996. The Regulations give the details about how the law should be applied.

I have supplied you with copies of all the relevant legislation that I considered when deciding upon your claim. (yes, all ten pages of them).

My decision is as follows:-

Date of claim 26/12/96

Mr S Turner, Mrs A Turner and their 3 dependent children are all members of the same household. (JSA Regulation 78 (1).

Mrs Turner had been temporarily absent from the household for a continuous period exceeding 4 weeks as at the date of claim. No allowance is therefore payable in respect of her. (JSA Regulations; Schedule 5; Column I, Paragraph 10).

Dependants allowances can be paid in respect of Daughters 1,2 and 3 for the first four weeks of their absence from the UK, commencing with the date of the claim to JSA (JSA Regulation 78 (5) (a) (i).

Any capital or income payable to a member of the family is treated as belonging to Mr Turner (JSA Regulation 88 (1) subject to certain disregards as outlined in Schedule 7 of the JSA Regulations. The Child Benefit paid to Mrs Turner is not subject to schedule 7.

Please do not hesitate to contact us if you need any further clarification of this decision.'

The key regulation was Regulation 78 (1) of the Jobseeker's Allowance Regulations which states:-

Subject to paragraphs (2) to (5), the claimant and any partner and, where the claimant and his partner is treated as responsible under Regulation 77 (circumstances in which a person is treated as responsible for another) for a child or young person, that child or young person and any child of that child or young person shall be treated for the purposes of the Act as members of the same household notwithstanding that any of them is temporarily living away from the other members of his family.'

Well that's clear enough although I would have thought that seven years away in France for the rest of the family constituted rather more than a temporary absence from England. Neither could any reasonable person consider that I was still part of the family as I had been away from them for over six months already and there was no guarantee that they would ever return from France.

Of course I didn't blame them personally. I had been a civil servant once and had received enough flack on the old Rating front to know that it was the law at fault, not the messenger. It is risible now but I can assure you that it was no laughing matter in early 1997. I had already seen my doctor again and he very kindly fixed me up with an appointment with a National Health counsellor. After listening to an hour's bile pouring out of me like a volcano, the counsellor subsequently sent me a letter calmly informing me that I wasn't suffering from clinical depression at all. What a fucking joke. The next little bad piece of news was a burglary by some gypsies at Heuré where Daughter No 2 lost a number of prized possessions. Worse still, Mandy's engagement ring that I had bought for her in Cape Town in 1975 had been stolen as well.

The Turner family now had their way at last. I had to go back to work. I had no choice to use my mother's parrot phrase. Of course I had a fucking choice. I could always revert to Plan B; to jump off the tower at Saint Gregory's church. Now that is what I would call perfect symmetry as I had also been married there over twenty one years ago. However of course I took the soft option as I hadn't the guts to actually finish myself off. So I went temping, starting by sorting out Mail Orders for some sort of flower power company in a grotty office in grotty North Street. I felt physically sick half the time but I fucking well did it. Next stop was a packing company putting together cardboard boxes and sticking numerous unmentionable items into them. At least the pay wasn't bad; £3.25 an hour. Roll on the Minimum Wage.

Finally, just before Easter I totally cracked after an apparently trivial incident with my mother. I just had to get away from Sudbury before the axe came out. I retreated in disarray up to Norfolk to stay with some old friends and to lick my wounds. They were a great comfort and eased me back on to the comeback trail. They also made the crucial suggestion that I should see a private counsellor. All this time my doctor had been supportive without actually diagnosing depression but suggested it might be a good idea for me to go on the pill; i.e. Prozac. I did so and have been taking it ever since. And that is why I am still alive. I then contacted a private counsellor as instructed and that's when I started to get down to what was really wrong at long, long last. As Kris Kristofferson wrote in his memorable song 'To Beat the Devil':-

'He nodded at my guitar and said: 'It's a tough life, isn't it?'
I just looked at him. He said: 'You ain't making much money, are you?'
I said: 'You've been reading my mail.'
He just smiled and said: ''Let me see that guitar.
I've got something you oughta hear.'
Then he laid it on me.

'If you waste your time a-talkin' to the people who don't listen.
To the things that you are sayin', who do you think's gonna hear.
And if you should die explainin' how the things that they complain about,
Are things they could be changin', who do you think's gonna care?'

Beating The Devil

Well, the old man was a stranger, but I'd heard his song before,
Back when failure locked me out on the other side of the door.
When no-one stood behind me but my shadow on the floor,
And lonesome was more than a state of mind.

You see, the devil haunts a hungry man,
If you don't wanna join him, you got to beat him.
I ain't saying I beat the devil, but I drank his beer for nothing,
And then I stole his song.'

Could I in turn 'Beat the Devil'?

Chapter 12 – Into the Mystic

> We were born before the wind
> Also younger than the sun
> Ere the bonnie boat was won
> As we sailed into the mystic
> Hark, now hear the sailors cry
> Smell the sea and feel the sky
> Let your soul and spirit fly into the mystic.

As usual Van was right on the money. My counsellor was brilliant as she went about the seemingly impossible task of repairing the mental and physical destruction. My new ally helped me to see that I didn't first run away from life in 1989 but in fact had been doing so since my sixth form at school, activated by a massive lack of self belief allied with an equal amount of self hate as 'shades of the prison house began to close on the growing boy'. This first manifested itself when I successfully launched a campaign of rebellion to avoid being captain of school rugby where I would then have to stand on stage before the whole school to dish out school colours. I had always been petrified of public speaking, and still am for that matter, or being on the stage at all. I now started to see that perhaps my life hadn't been a total failure and I hadn't wasted those seven long years in France. It was just all part of life's rich experience.

> 'Sorrow is knowledge: they who know the most
> Must mourn the deepest o'er the fatal truth
> The Tree of Knowledge is not that of life.'

Equally important I learnt to forgive myself and to forgive others; notably my parents. This helped to release me from the shackles of my past so that I could now go forward and to use that corny old cliché, unlock my potential. At the same time I started to perceive my blessings in non-material terms. For some reason Mandy hadn't yet driven a carving knife into my hunched back, although that was of course the main reason I had returned to England to severely limit her opportunities. I also had the great fortune to have three beautiful and talented daughters. How could a man so ugly on the inside and outside be so lucky?

On the work front I had now moved on to Tollman's Engineering putting toilet cleaners into little packets. I had no idea before that the Great British Public inserted so many funny objects down their U bends. However here I began if not to actually enjoy the work, to use two words that was im-possible, but to enjoy the camaraderie. My co-workers were a friendly crew if that isn't too condescending, and were quick to assist me and my fumbling fingers. Christ, I was crap even in the bog business, but again gave myself a few points for sticking it out. But how could anyone endure this mental drudgery for over seven years and remain cheerful, like the girl working next to me, I couldn't begin to fathom. However I did start to comprehend that a minimum wage of £4 an hour was neither greedy or inflationary. Consequently I realized that I was ambivalent about returning to the fat cats of the property world. Me, a so-called middle class workshy snob, was at last learning the walk of life. I was also in the right place at the right time to celebrate that gloriously sunny May 1st, 1997 when that nice John Major and his dwindling band of Tories, in the original totally unflattering sense of the word, finally met their electoral Armageddon. What a defeat. The oily Portillo, the grasping Mellor and Mr and Mrs smelling of roses Hamilton all gone. What a feeling! It was almost as good as sex. No, on second thoughts it was much, much better. It was a kind of indefinite spiritual orgasm.

I had now earned enough money to go out and visit the family again in France and this time it went a lot more satisfactorily. I also unearthed the original documents authenticating the price and proof of purchase of Mandy's engagement ring in Cape Town and we went together to see the insurance agent in Auch. He appeared satisfied with the documentation and said that we would be paid the maximum figure under the policy of twenty five thousand francs within two to three weeks, *'pas de problème'*. Whenever you hear that latter phrase you should always be on your guard but at the time I wasn't in listening mode. But as soon as Mandy and the family had safely returned to England and out of the way the insurance agent reneged on his agreement and even threatening solicitor's letters elucidated no joy. So now Monsieur Ducassé of Concorde Assurance, stand up and take a bow, your past has finally caught up with you.

Back from the sunny South West of France, it was on to job number four at the infamous Bakers Mill. From the sublime to the slime you might say. The job was packing cat and dog biscuits and the smell was almost as distinctive as that of the Westgate Brewery or the sugar beet factory at Bury Saint Edmunds, if slightly less perfumed. I was employed mostly in the stacking and wrapping of various sized boxes which although terminally boring, was infinitely preferable to the fiddly and quickfire process of packing. Here the conveyor belt surged at you relentlessly for up to two hours for a time. I just couldn't keep up with all those bloody biscuits. Again I asked myself where had it all gone wrong? What was a middle-aged Chartered Surveyor doing in this place? I suppose that chilling out was the correct answer. I was chatting to a fellow worker there one day and speculated who was the most brain dead person in the establishment. His answer was illuminating.

'Do you know, I have often wondered the same thing myself.'

It certainly helped to be a little lacking there or better still, to have a hyperactive sense of humour. Funnily enough having completed my stint there I felt a real sense of achievement. It was certainly the hardest I had ever worked physically in my life. All the other temps who had started at the same time as me had fallen by the wayside for one reason or another and I was the only one left standing by the end of my temporary contract. I was also horrified by the amount of racism there and vowed never to darken the door of Bakers Mill again. Happily I have kept that promise. Even better the old factory has recently been demolished to be replaced by some 'superbly situated' riverside houses and flats. It also helped that England had a great win over the Aussies in the Ist Test at Edgbaston whilst I was at Bakers Mill. As I have said before never underestimate the power of sport to aid the old feel good factor. Luckily I was well away from there when we got comprehensively derailed later in the series.

Suddenly the feel good factor was very good indeed. First Mandy found a buyer for Heuré and the preliminary contract was soon signed despite the usual last minute alarms. Completion was fixed for late August.

Secondly I won my appeal in late June against the Benefits Agency on an obscure technicality under the selfsame Section 78 of the jolly old Jobseekers Allowances Regulations 1996. I had done it by reading the good old small print again, this time to more positive effect, and the result was a technical knockout. I defeated the Benefits Agency on the vital Paragraph (2) (b) of the Regulations which stated as follows:-

(2) Paragraph (1) shall not apply to a person who is living away from the other members of his family where –

(a) That person does not intend living with the other members of his family;

Or

(b)   His absence from the other members of the family is likely to exceed 52 weeks, unless there are exceptional circumstances (for example the person is in hospital or otherwise has no control over the length of his absence), and the absence is unlikely to be substantially more than 52 weeks.

I argued that that I should be treated as a single person under the regulations as my absence was certain to exceed 52 weeks because it was not financially possible for my family to move back to England until they had received the proceeds from the sale of the house. I went on to say that:-

'Even if I sold my house subject to contract tomorrow it would be impossible under French law to complete in under 3 months because after the 'Acte Definitive' is signed the Notaire has to then get clearance from the Bureau de Hypothèques before he can release any money.'

Of course between the time of my appeal and the Tribunal's decision we had in fact sold Heuré and I am afraid I was a little bit economical with the truth here. However the Tribunal were in no position to dispute my interpretation of French law, they had more than enough law on their plate with the fiendish Jobseekers Regulations in England.

As a local firm of solicitors, the Citizens Advice Bureau and the Royal Institution of Chartered Surveyors had all in their triumviratal wisdom advised me that I hadn't got a case, my personal pleasure was childishly unconfined and the boost to my self confidence atomic, plus the considerable financial bonus that my Jobseekers Allowance was to be back-dated to February.

That's the trouble with being a tormented genius. One is either effortlessly superior to most of the human race or pathetically below them. There is no half way house for him. I think that perhaps I have still a little way to go with my shrink.

However having won my case I couldn't mention depression as I would then be unavailable for work. If I was mentally ill I wasn't entitled to Jobseekers Allowance but if I did fuck all and pretended to be sane then I was. A classic Catch 22 if ever I saw one. Yossarian would have been very proud of that piece of legislation.

Thirdly I doubled my mother's pension. I should explain that since Dad's death she was now entitled to a War Widow's pension again as her first husband had been killed in the war. This involved a long visit to the Records Office in London to trace his death certificate. I also found out at the same time that he had died at Manston airfield in Kent where I had unwittingly run my sole marathon ten years earlier.

Fourthly Chris Vos and SAFER had finally sold a farm to a Mr Warrilow, a former client, and had sent Mandy a cheque for nineteen thousand nine hundred francs. The full commission was twenty thousand francs but Chris had deducted precisely one hundred francs on account of a green fee I had failed to pay for him at Fleurance eighteen months earlier. I had introduced this client to Chris after only minimum output from me, apart from on the golf course of course. Talk about swings and roundabouts, adversity certainly shows who your true friends are. *C'est normal* said Chris. Oh no it wasn't and but it certainly shows that somebody up there moves in mysterious ways.

Talking of the deity the sessions with my counsellor had taken off my intellectual blinkers as I finally turned a questioning mind to religion and started to reverse all those barren years of brainwashing.

'What can this Gospel of Jesus be?
What life and immortality
What was that he brought to light
That Plato and Cicero did not write?'

And good old Omar Khayyam was on the money as usual.

'And do you think that unto such as you
A maggot-minded, starved, fanatic crew
God gave a secret, and denied it me?
Well, well – what matters it? Believe that, too!'

But perhaps the most erudite and elegant demolition of Christianity came in Edward Gibbon's famous Chapter XV of his imperious work 'The Decline and Fall of the Roman Empire'. He concludes Chapter XV as follows:-

'But how shall we excuse the supine inattention of the Pagan and philosophic world, to those evidences which were presented by the hand of Omnipotence, not to their reason, but to their senses? During the age of Christ, of his apostles, and of their first disciples, the doctrine which they preached was confirmed by innumerable prodigies. The lame walked, the blind saw, the sick were healed, the dead were raised, demons were expelled, and the laws of nature were frequently suspended for the benefit of the church. But the sages of Greece and Rome turned aside from the awful spectacle, and pursuing the ordinary occupations of life and study, appeared unconscious of any alterations in the moral or physical government of the world. Under the reign of Tiberius, the whole earth, or at least a celebrated province of the Roman empire, was involved in a praeternatural darkness of three hours. Even this miraculous event, which ought to have excited the wonder, the curiosity, and the devotion of mankind, passed without notice in an age of science and history. It happened during the lifetime of Seneca and the elder

Pliny, who must have experienced the immediate effects, or received the earliest intelligence, of the prodigy. Each of these philosophers, in a laborious work, has recorded all the great phenomena of nature, earthquakes, meteors, comets, and eclipses, which his indefatigable curiosity could collect. Both the one and the other have omitted to mention the greatest phenomenon to which the mortal eye has been witness since the creation of the globe. A distinct chapter of Pliny is designed for eclipses of an extraordinary nature and unusual duration; but he contents himself with describing the singular defect of light which followed the murder of Caesar, when, during the greatest part of a year, the orb appeared pale and without splendour. This season of obscurity, which cannot surely be compared with the praeternatural darkness of the Passion, had already been celebrated by most of the poets and historians of that memorable age.'

Any of you out there still with an open mind on the subject of religion might read with profit 'The Importance of Living' by that great pagan Lin Yutang. Here is a poem from the Great Book.

'So then, at heart, I feel I'm half a Buddha,
And almost half a Taoist fairy blest.
One half myself to Father heaven I
Return: the other half to children leave-'

The true halfway house for those with peace of mind.

Back to the more mundane task of paying the bills. Mum had continued to support me all this time to carry on in Dad's best tradition of bailing me out as and when financial disaster beckoned, but more from her own maternal and Christian love, whereas I still had the continuous battle of relating finances to philosophy. Our two approaches just didn't gel. In spite of my turning away from faith just as my father had, Mum remained a good and devout Christian all her life and drew great comfort from it, as does Mandy. Each to his own.

Money in the bank hadn't helped me when I first moved to Heuré and it wasn't going to help now. I just had to win the mind game against depression. Prozac certainly helped a lot against the massive mood swings but its beneficial effects were greatly diluted by alcohol. Because of the colossal fall in the franc against the pound in the previous year we were going to lose the little matter of twenty thousand francs in currency depreciation when Heuré was finally sold. On the other hand all Mandy's improvements more than saw off this loss. When I reflect upon this I still find it sad that Monsieur *Je ne regrette rien* Lamont couldn't muster an itsy bitsy apology when he lost over four billion in a single day on that very Black Wednesday in 1993. Oh silly me, I forgot, it was all the fault of that nasty Mr Soros. Then Mr L was elevated to the House of Lords for his troubles. What a system.

However I was still resolved to buy a house in England especially when I found out I would need more references, which of course I would never obtain now, just to rent a property. It meant I wouldn't have any cash left over for starting up the property search company and I also had to be rather parsimonious with the truth with the lending company with one of those now discredited Self Certificated mortgage applications. In fact let's not beat about the bush, I told the company a load of pork pies. Luckily the mortgage is safely paid off so I trust I am now in the clear. Ironically this house proved to be one of my best buys as the market took off into orbit again soon after we purchased it. As for the property search company it was in any event ten years too late for that project in retrospect and it would have been doomed to failure again. If I was going to set one up I should have done it in 1989 when I had the capital instead of buggering off to France.

Ah hindsight, whatever would we do without it?

Enfin, having spent a long and lonely year away from Mandy and the girls, they returned from France shortly after the signing in late August. However Mandy had made it quite clear that whilst living in France she realized she would have to sell her dream house before she could divorce and that could still happen. It had been an interesting year but not one to be repeated on a regular basis and, most surprisingly, Mandy and the family stayed.

'For those who going through the vale of misery use it as a well, these pools are filled with water, but also with pearls of great price and buried treasure, and I have been blessed to find them.'

That is true serendipity.

It was very strange to be together again and not all of the brood were happy to be back in England to put it mildly. In fact they hadn't asked to go to France and hadn't asked to come back either. It is a miracle they still talk to me. Daughter No 3 had been only four when she left England and had first learnt to read and write in French. As she had subsequently spent two thirds of her life in France she considered she was far more French than English. Daughter No 2 was almost as ambivalent whilst Daughter No 1, who had refused to speak a word to anyone on the long journey back to England, was later more philosophical when she found a *copain* (boy friend) in London and Sudbury train station was online for Liverpool Street, so to speak. The other problem was that Mandy had to leave her beloved Paddy in the dog pound because she couldn't even contemplate putting him through the inhuman quarantine system then prevailing. Of course the magnificent Passport for Pets campaign didn't actually achieve its abolition until 2001. In fact I only just picked up Mandy's vote over Paddy but Mum again couldn't understand that everyone has a choice in life and dogs don't suffer from alcoholism or depression as far as I know. Mum just didn't get it. Mandy didn't have to come back with the children. They had managed very well in France once they had got rid of me and it was a damn close run thing in the end, how close I didn't realize at the time.

Our first weekend together found us at R and B's cottage near The National Trust's Blickling Hall near Aylesham some miles north of Norwich. We were having a gentle lie-in idly listening to the radio when we realized they seemed to be talking rather obsessively about Diana, Princess of Wales. Then we realized they were talking about her in the past tense. Then the whole, bizarre story unfolded through the course of the morning. I am afraid I wasn't a great fan of Diana but what a tragedy to die so young and again 'what a stupid way to die'. Like an awful number of people I will always connect that exact moment and place with the news of her death.

We all had to stay a further three months with Mum which put a further strain on family relationships all round. Finally we thankfully moved into a modern but modest house in Chianti Court in late October despite our solicitor having some difficulty in identifying who he was acting for.

Away from the house the girls were settling in well back at an English school although they naturally found a lot of things very strange, uniforms for one and accents another. Who was this strange foreigner called Geoffrey Boycox or some such unpronounceable name? Although their spoken English was *pas mal* their actual experience of writing the language was limited to thank you letters.

On the work front I was still trying to sell articles to national newspapers and magazines but they weren't falling over themselves to sign me up. Mandy was doing a much longer stint than me on the packing front to pay for a training course at college, but then again she wasn't constrained by such English niceties as snobbery and philosophy. Then in desperation I applied for a job with

Waitrose as a Car Park Assistant but the young whippersnapper who subsequently interviewed me thought I was possibly overqualified. I then applied for another job with Coral Bookmakers as a Cashier. My job application letter started promisingly and rather wittily, even if I say so myself:

'Accordingly I find myself financially gelded at the moment to utilize a spot of racing
parlance and am 'available for work' again, to borrow Henry Longhurst's immortal phrase.'

And then I went and spoilt it all by continuing:

'To change the subject for a moment I note with interest your policy on Equal Opportunities. Having studied the small print it would appear to be OK if I am a one-armed homosexual Mormon Irishman of Black Caribbean origin, but not OK if I am an ordinary agnostic married Englishman of a certain age. Please correct me if I am mistaken.'

Funnily enough, I didn't get the job. Perhaps they thought I would put my hand in the till, but Daughter No 2 now uses this letter as an example of how not to write a job application. I was so arrogant even when my self-esteem was zero. This is what a mental health problem does to you. You just lose all sense of judgement and common sense.

I had then one final abortive sally into the property world with a nondescript local firm before they decided I was rather nondescript as well and gave me the push. I therefore retired from the property world very, very hurt for definitely the final time. Yesterday's gone: sans Valuation Office, sans Hamptons and sans *promeneurs*. Yeeeeees. My father couldn't have been more right.

I also had all the time in the world to confront the demon drink. I finally admitted to myself and to Mandy that I was an alcoholic and had been *depuis longtemps*. However what I don't admit is all that crap about once an alcoholic, always an alcoholic. To hell with Alcoholics Anonymous and their insidious brand of brainwashing. Alcoholism is a temporary illness like depression, not a terminal one. *On verra, pas un verre*, is my new motto although the situation isn't ameliorated by Sebastian Faulks' wry observation that a writer needs 'slightly more (income) to live on. He apparently needs to drink more alcohol.'

On the work front I am still not making much money but I have now found something else much more important and it's called soul. Play it again Van:-

'Turn it up, that's enough, so you know it's got soul.'

Talking about not making much money, a few years ago there was a brilliant article on the subject by that fine journalist and author Howard Jacobson 'It is a chilling thought, but the proof of good writing does not lie in the reading'. In it Jacobson wrote about three sentences he had just happened upon and wished he had written. These three sentences (by Ford Maddox Ford) are as follows:-

'For myself, I care nothing about readers for writers. It is sufficient that the book should be on the shelf or the manuscript, down the years slowly gathering the infiltrated dust out of the bottom of the chest, indeed it is enough that the words making it up should have ever been gathered together beneath a pen Force once created is indestructible: we may let it go at that. Or the manuscript.'

As Jacobson comments. 'Mark that. Or the manuscript. Meaning that in the end, taking the long view, it might not matter a fig to anything but the author's bank balance, which is no consideration whatsoever, whether his words make it into book form at all.

But we are children of an age unable to measure anything except by the laws of marketing. Nothing is valuable for itself. A book must have its readers because a writer must have his money. And only when he has money can his work be accounted a success.'

So as Jacobson concludes. 'Almost nobody has read this novel – that's what I would like to see more of on book jackets. Read this – no one else has, would be better. And best of all. Suit yourself – the writer is indifferent to your curiosity or opinion, and writes only for writing's sake.

Then we would be getting back to what we are supposed to be about.'

But perhaps Howard has changed his mind now that he has gone and spoilt it all by recently winning the Big Daddy of the book prize world, the Man Booker, and subsequently seen the sales of 'The Finkler Question' soar into orbit.

So there we have it.

'And when the foghorn blows you know I will be coming home
And when the foghorn whistle blows I got to hear it
I don't have to fear it
And I want to rock your gypsy soul
Just like in the days of old
And magnificently we will flow into the mystic
Come on girl......'

It's too late to stop now, isn't it?

EPILOGUE: DECEMBER 2010

Thirteen years later it is finally all over and the feel good factor is still very good indeed. England have just retained the Ashes 'Down Under' to keep our minds off the bitterly cold weather in the UK. However whilst we are on the cricket front I must take this opportunity of confessing to the mortal sin of failing the 'Tebbut Test' *de temps en temps*. Age is obviously withering me as I don't seem to care very much these days if England win any more; I just like watching good Test Match cricket. In fact I would dare to go much further and venture that another England collapse like at Perth signifies everything is normal and all is well with the world in this best of all possible worlds, but when England start winning consistently there is danger at the door. So long live Test cricket and long live England collapses. Anyway cricket doesn't <u>really</u> matter at the end of the day, does it?

On the work front I have finally made a little money, but 'On the Road' as a Private Hire Driver for six hard years, and not as a writer. I have also written and published two books, neither of which made any money. To continue consistently in this vein, I therefore present this little memoir not with the hope it will bring me a fortune (but as with Howard Jacobson's post 'Finkler' stance I wouldn't say no to a modest pension to support me in my more mature years) but with the fervent hope that it brings a modicum of comfort and help to some of those thousands of people out there who either have suffered or are still suffering from 'The Devil'. I must stress that it <u>is</u> possible to beat depression, or what Lewis Wolpert poignantly called the 'Malignant Sadness', and what I more prosaically call 'The Devil'. Play it again Kris:-

'I ain't saying I beat the devil
But I drank his beer for nothing.'

And I am still drinking it with a little help from my friends.

One thing I was especially pleased with was that I had a total reconciliation with my mother before her death three years ago, appropriately on the night following Mothering Sunday. Only in January on her 89th birthday she had declared that 'old age is a bugger' and she wasn't going to live till 90. She fulfilled that wish and died gently in the night. She had been ill for some time and I am delighted that I managed to help her just a little bit in those last declining years. We had the funeral at Saint Gregory's Church where Mandy and I got married over thirty one years ago. Mum wanted it to be a Service of Thanksgiving ('not a sad affair') to all her family and friends whose love had made it such a good life. In that spirit she had selected as one of the hymns the spirited and uplifting 'The Lord of the Dance', then 'Lord of all Hopefulness, Lord of all Joy' and finally the intensely moving 'The Day Thou Gavest is Ended'. Canon Arthur Dunlop gave a fine eulogy and I finished by reading the poem 'I Did Not Die' that my niece Alice had sent to Mum when Dad died and which she had found so poignant at the time.

'Do not stand at my grave and weep.
I am not there. I do not sleep.

I am a thousand winds that blow;
I am the diamond glints on snow.
I am the sunlight on ripened grain;
I am the gentle Autumn's rain.

I am in the morning hush
I am in the graceful rush
Of beautiful birds in circling flight,
I am the starshine of the night.

I am in the flowers that bloom,
I am in a quiet room.
I am in the birds that sing,

I am in each lovely thing.

Do not stand at my grave and cry
I am not there. I did not die.'

By an incredibly sad co-incidence Canon Dunlop died of a heart attack the very same evening after Mum's service and we were back at his Saint Gregory's for his funeral exactly a week later. In fact I have now completed Four Funerals and a Wedding there. The third funeral was my dear old friend David Francis who died of stomach cancer at the age of only fifty eight. Dave had been best man at my wedding and we had been through a lot together. We had driven a Land Rover from Algiers to Cape Town in 1973/4 and then stayed on in Cape Town subsequently meeting both our future wives there.   One indelible memory of our carefree youth was sharing a joint together during 'The Trip' on Nyali Beach near Mombasa at midnight while listening to 'Have you seen the stars tonight?' by the legendary Jefferson Airplane. We certainly did that night Dave. The fourth funeral was of Doreen who had worked for Mum for many years and when I was only three, had rescued my right arm which had got stuck in the ringer used to dry washing in the primitive early fifties. I still bear the scar to this day but Doreen certainly saved me from a much more severe injury. The wedding in question after all those funerals was for 'baby' Daughter No 3 two years ago.

Mandy is still miraculously with me, the girls are all thriving in their chosen endeavours and I am so proud of them after their unconventional and unsettling upbringing. As mentioned above Daughter No 3 got married in 2008 and with delicious irony or deadly intent her new husband is a Tax Consultant, but a very nice guy despite it. I think she has made a very wise choice. The wedding was in mid September and it turned into a magical autumnal day as the sun broke through just before the service and shone brightly down on proceedings for the rest of the day.

Daughter No 3 looked radiant, Daughters 1 and 2 were the glamorous bridesmaids and I managed to avoid tripping over while escorting the bride nervously up the aisle. All things were certainly bright and beautiful as the first hymn said. Bill Crawte richly read those lyrical words from First Corinthians 13.

'Love is patient; love is kind and envies no one. Love is never boastful, nor conceited, nor rude; never selfish, not quick to take offence. Love keeps no score of wrongs; does not gloat over other men's sins, but delights in the truth. There is nothing love cannot face; there is no limit to its faith, its hope, and its endurance.'

Finally Helen Brooker read from Captain Corelli's Mandolin.

'Love is a temporary madness. It erupts like an earthquake and then subsides. And when it subsides you have to make a decision. You have to workout whether your roots have become so entwined together that is inconceivable that you should ever part. Because this is what love is. Love is not breathfulness, it is not excitement, it is not the promulgation of promises of eternal passion. That is just being 'in love' which any of us can convince ourselves we are.

Love itself is what is left over when being in love has burned away, and this both an art and a fortunate accident. Your mother and I had it, we had roots that grew towards each other underground, and when all the pretty blossom had fallen from the branches we found we were one tree and not two.'

Wonderful words and beautifully spoken. Truly a wonderful day as well. Tragically Helen is gravely ill as I write this. After all the trials and tribulations she had been through in her younger days, she had battled through to make a real success of her life, only to be struck down in her prime. Life is so bloody unfair at times, as is death.

After the May General Election the whole country was looking forward to the exciting prospect of the first coalition government for sixty five years after the fourteen sorry years of New Labour under Blair and Brown. But could the new government bring Britain new hope? The jury is obviously still out on that one but already there are worrying signs of fissure and failure, not only on the economic front but more worrying on foreign fields.

Talking about new hope, over four decades of independence have brought little cause for optimism in Algeria recent years. As Sir Alistair Horne wrote in his 2006 Preface to 'A Savage War of Peace':

'Over half a century has passed since that All Saint's Day in the Aurès Mountains, historic for Algeria, dreadful for France, when two young French schoolteachers on their honeymoon, the Monnerots, were hauled off their bus and shot down. That is a long time in modern memory. Yet this story of how a handful of Algerian guerrillas, primitively armed, but masterfully deploying the weapon of terror, outwitted and out-fought over eight years the best armies that France could provide, remains on the statute books as a prototype of the modern war of national liberation. In South Africa the ANC studied it carefully, prior to the release and apotheosis of Nelson Mandela; in their unleashing of intifada against Israel, Palestinian leaders have looked ardently towards it. So has al-Qaeda. Since the events of September 11, 2001, the west has needed to take a new, hard look at Algeria's 'Savage War of Peace', and all that has flowed from it.'

At many times the peace in Algeria has been no less savage than the war, and the 1990's introduced the cruel influence of Islamic fundamentalism across the land. Starting with the killing of local policemen, just as in 1954, an appalling civil war ensued with the return of the infamous' Kabyle smile' (throat slitting). The FIS (Islamic Salvation Front) was thrust aside by a far more extreme band of revolutionaries, the GIA (Armed Islam Group) prepared to wage war with total ruthlessness. Its origins and leaders were surrounded by mystery, but its aims appeared to be projected towards a complete and anarchic destruction of the existing order. On a note that was to become pointedly obvious on September 11th, 2001, some of its killers were known as the 'Afghans', highly trained volunteers who had served their apprenticeship in that country. By the end of 2001 another 100,000 Algerians had been slaughtered.

In France the civil war between Algerians of the 1990's overflowed across the Mediterranean. On Christmas Eve 1994 Air France Flight 8969 was hijacked at Algiers airport by the GIA with 220 passengers and 12 flight crew on board. By the end of Christmas Day three passengers had been shot dead and another 63 released. On Boxing Day the pilot of the plane was eventually allowed to take off for Marseille, where it was due to refuel before continuing on to Paris. However in Marseille the hijackers requested that 27 tonnes of fuel being put in, even though the plane only need 9-10 tonnes to fly to Paris. The request confirmed to the French authorities from prior intelligence that the plane was going to be used as a missile on a suicide attack on the centre of Paris itself. This forced the hand of the authorities and the French Prime Minister Édouard Balladur gave permission for Major Denis Favier, the head of the Groupe d'Intervention de la Gendarmerie National (GIGN), to take whatever actions he felt were necessary. After the hijackers opened fire on the control tower, Favier decided to act. The raid was both daring and incredibly successful, with all the remaining passengers and crew escaping alive, while the four hijackers were all killed. The crew of the A300 and the GIGN forces all received national honours. A former militant group leader later admitted that the hijackers had planned to detonate the aircraft over the

Eiffel Tower. Of course America and the rest of the world conveniently forgot about Flight 8969 until the September 11th attack on the Twin Towers in 2001almost seven years later.

Then in 1995 and 1996 feuding between rival clans of the GIA brought terrorism to the Paris Metro, of which I was an unwilling spectator on my abortive trip up north to see the Great Dane, killing and wounding over eighty people. Again did America take any notice of a little terrorism outside its own back yard at the time? No, of course it didn't. When Blair and Bush went blindly into both Iraq and Afghanistan, at the same time inflaming the Arab world, a prior study of the Algerian War might have made them think twice, thrice or even four times.

More than anything, they might have learnt that the use of torture was ultimately one of the cardinal reasons for the defeat in Algeria, as Frenchmen realised that methods of interrogation were being used similar to those during the Nazi occupation. As Horne also wrote:-

'As a further footnote to my tenet, learned in Algeria, that torture should never, never, never be resorted to by any Western society. I draw readers once again to the testimony of Prefect Teitgen of Algiers which – three decades on – I still find deeply moving. Teitgen had been informed by the Algiers police that they had intelligence of a bomb which could have caused appalling casualties. Could they put a suspect to 'the question?' Himself a deportee in World War 2, Teitgen told me he refused:

........I trembled the whole afternoon. Finally the bomb did not go off. Thank God I was right. Because if you once get into the torture business, you're lost.......All our so-called civilisation is covered with a varnish. Scratch it, and underneath you find fear.....When you see the throats of your *copains* slit, then the varnish disappears.

How applicable this still is to the dilemmas facing the west in the War on Terror!'

Back to more prosaic domestic issues. I'm still on 'The Pill'. I have tried to come off it on several occasions whenever I thought I felt really OK. However on each occasion I slid inexorably back into depression after the effects of the Seriotonin gradually worked its way out of my system. Now I am on strict instructions from Mandy to keep taking it for life. She argues quite reasonably that it doesn't really matter if there are any delayed side effects as without it I would either be dead already or she would certainly have left me. Long live Prozac and bugger 'The Devil'!

But as Elizabeth Wurtzel wrote in Prozac Nation:-

'The secret I sometimes think that only I know is that Prozac really isn't that great. Of course I can say this and still believe that Prozac was the miracle that saved my life and jump-started me out of a full-time state of depression – which would probably seem to most people reason enough to think of the drug as manna from heaven. But after six years on Prozac, I know that it is not the end but the beginning. Mental health is so much more complicated than any pill that any mortal could invent.'

The battle wages continuously and I keep asking myself if this book is another 'failure' am I still a failure? Alas, unlike Dylan, it is for me to decide.

'Does any doctor prescribe landscape nowadays? Until recently, for certain ailments of body and mind, tuberculosis or depression, it was all that could be prescribed. There are, wrote Richard Jefferies, 'three potent medicines of nature', the sea, the air and the sun. And he might have added the scenes which these elements both created and contain, for if anyone set out for a thorough, self-prescribed landscape cure, he did.'

So wrote the distinguished Suffolk writer Ronald Blythe in his chapter Remedial Scenes from Second Nature (1984). I too have taken solace in the landscape cure first in gentle Suffolk and then in the shape of the formidable 630 mile South West Coast Path which I finally finished this summer and am now the proud new record holder of the slowest ever time to complete (forty one years, *pas mal hein*?).

'Once again
Do I behold these steep and lofty cliffs,
That on a wild secluded scene impress
Thoughts of more deep seclusion: and connect
The landscape with the quiet of the sky.'

Thanks again Mr Wordsworth.

So there you have it. Keep taking 'The Pill' and keep on walking.

Now if you will excuse me the long day's task is done and I am going to seek out Lawrence Durrell's immortal 'Tree of Idleness' at Bellapaix and have a little lie down. I think I have just about earned it by now.

Lightning Source UK Ltd.
Milton Keynes UK

175848UK00001B/30/P